The essential
researcher's handbook
2002.

www.harcourt-international.com

Bringing you products from all Harcourt Health Sciences companies including Baillière Tindall, Churchill Livingstone, Mosby and W.B. Saunders

- ▷ **Browse** for latest information on new books, journals and electronic products

- ▷ **Search** for information on over 20 000 published titles with full product information including tables of contents and sample chapters

- ▷ **Keep up to date** with our extensive publishing programme in your field by registering with eAlert or requesting postal updates

- ▷ **Secure online ordering** with prompt delivery, as well as full contact details to order by phone, fax or post

- ▷ **News** of special features and promotions

If you are based in the following countries, please visit the country-specific site to receive full details of product availability and local ordering information

USA: www.harcourthealth.com

Canada: www.harcourtcanada.com

Australia: www.harcourt.com.au

❧ Baillière Tindall   ⚓ CHURCHILL LIVINGSTONE   Ⓜ Mosby   Ⓦ W.B. SAUNDERS

The Essential Researcher's Handbook

About the Editors

Maggie Tarling (née Bolger) is now an Integrated Care Pathways Coordinator, following five years' experience as a Senior Research Nurse in anaesthetics and a brief spell as a lecturer for the ENB182 course at Thames Valley University. She did her nurse training at the Central Middlesex Hospital in 1982 and midwifery at the Royal Berkshire Hospital in 1984. She spent most of her nursing career in operating theatres. In 1992, she completed a BSc (Hons) in Psychology at the London Guildhall University and in 1994 an MSc in Health Psychology at City University. She has published and presented many papers in anaesthetics and ITU. She was part of the research team that researched the impact of an ITU outreach team. This has been recognised by the Department of Health as a model of best practice for critically ill patients.

Linda Crofts (née Fennell) is Course Leader at the Health and Social Services Institute, University of Essex, where she divides her time between teaching, research and consultancy to local NHS Trusts. As part of this diverse role she is Research and Development Adviser to Local Health Partnerships NHS Trust in Suffolk. She previously worked as Director of Nursing Research and Development at Barts and the London NHS Trust, a post she held for over 5 years. She is a qualified Nurse Teacher and held various teaching posts at the Royal Free Hospital, where she also trained as a Registered General Nurse and later developed a career in operating theatre nursing. She recently completed the Kings Fund/Johnson and Johnson Nursing Leadership programme and now uses much of the learning through this in undertaking 'whole systems' work.

For Baillière Tindall:

Senior Commissioning Editor: Sarena Wolfaard
Project Development Manager: Mairi McCubbin
Project Manager: Jane Dingwall
Designer: Judith Wright

The Essential Researcher's Handbook

for Nurses and Health Care Professionals

Edited by

Maggie Tarling BSc MSc RGN RM

Integrated Care Pathways Coordinator, University Hospital Lewisham, London, UK

Linda Crofts BA(Hons) MSc DipNEd RGN RNT

Health and Social Services Institute, University of Essex, Colchester, UK

Foreword by

Alison Kitson DPhil RN FRCN

Director, RCN Institute, London, UK

SECOND EDITION

BAILLIÈRE TINDALL
Edinburgh London New York Philadelphia St Louis Sydney Toronto 2002

BAILLIÈRE TINDALL An imprint of Harcourt Publishers Limited

© Baillière Tindall 1998
© Harcourt Publishers Limited 2002

is a registered trademark of Harcourt Publishers Limited

The right of Maggie Tarling and Linda Crofts to be identified as editors of this work has been asserted by them in accordance with the Copyright, Designs and Patents Act 1988

First edition 1998
Second edition 2002

ISBN 0 7020 2636 0

British Library Cataloguing in Publication Data
A catalogue record for this book is available from the British Library

Library of Congress Cataloging in Publication Data
A catalog record for this book is available from the Library of Congress

Note
Medical knowledge is constantly changing. As new information becomes available, changes in treatment, procedures, equipment and the use of drugs become necessary. The editors, contributors and the publishers have taken care to ensure that the information given in this text is accurate and up to date. However, readers are strongly advised to confirm that the information, especially with regard to drug usage, complies with the latest legislation and standards of practice.

The
publisher's
policy is to use
**paper manufactured
from sustainable forests**

Printed in China

Contents

Contributors

Sandra Colville-Stewart BSc BSN PhD RGN RN ALA
Research Sister, MRC Bright Study, Clinical
Pharmacology, St. Bartholomew's Medical School,
London, UK
3. *How to do a Literature Search*

Linda Crofts BA(Hons) MSc DipNEd RGN RNT
Health and Social Services Institute,
University of Essex, Colchester, UK
1. *Getting Started*
2. *The Context of Research in the NHS*
4. *Reviewing the Literature*
6. *Writing a Proposal*
9. *Venturing into the Field*
10. *Reporting Results*

Joan Curzio BSc MSc PhD RGN
Project Leader, Nursing Research Initiative for
Scotland, Faculty of Health, Glasgow Caledonian
University, Glasgow, UK
7. *Research Funding*

Joyce E. Kenkre MSc RGN
Professor of Primary Care, School of Care Sciences,
University of Glamorgan, Pontypridd, UK
12. *Careers in Research*

Jill E. Robinson BSc PhD RMN CertEd ILTM
Centre for Applied Research in Education, School of
Education and Professional Development, University
of East Anglia, Norwich, UK
5. *Choosing your Methods*

Maggie Tarling BSc MSc RGN RM
Integrated Care Pathways Coordinator, University
Hospital Lewisham, London, UK
6. *Writing a Proposal*
8. *Ethical Issues*
9. *Venturing into the Field*
10. *Reporting Results*
11. *Disseminating Research Findings*

Foreword

The lifeblood of any practice discipline resides in its ability to generate, refine, and continuously test out new knowledge. Such a commitment is a hallmark of professional practice and ensures the protection of both patients and professionals themselves.

Instead of being an optional extra, the approach to researching our practice should therefore be right at the heart of the way we think. The clinical skills we spend years refining – accurate observation, logical analysis, drawing on and analysing diverse sources of evidence, using our intuition, reflecting critically on our practice and disciplining ourselves to evaluate the impact of our practice on patient care – these are all essential skills in the armoury of beginning researchers. If this excites and energises you, then you are ready for more: more tools and techniques that will help you shift from everyday problem-solving and clinical evaluation (that aids audit and clinical governance) to more complex problem-solving and research approaches.

Maggie Tarling and Linda Crofts have produced a very accessible and helpful guide to this process. It should be rewarding and fun; it will certainly require persistence, thoroughness, open-mindedness and a good dollop of determination. In fact, all those skills required to be a successful health professional. The reward is manifold: through improving your research skills you will also be reinforcing improved ways of thinking about your professional practice, and that must surely be good for patient care.

London, 2001   Alison Kitson

Preface

It gives us great pleasure to present the second edition of this book. Since the first edition there have been sweeping changes in the National Health Service. With the launch of 'clinical governance' there has been an increased need to ensure that our practice is evidence based. There have also been fundamental changes in the way research is funded and managed within the NHS, with a focus on a responsibility for research governance. With the introduction of the Human Rights Act, legal requirements may, for the first time, have an impact on how research will be conducted. We also have a greater access to information on the internet, and an increase in the use of information technology (IT) in our daily practice. We have endeavoured to include and review these changes in this edition.

However, some things do not change and our focus is still upon the practicalities of conducting research. In order to gain the most from the book, it is important that the reader has some understanding of research methodologies and good clinical practice guidelines. There are many excellent research textbooks on the market; these should be used in conjunction with this book, which focuses on the day-to-day practicalities of 'doing research'.

London, 2001   Maggie Tarling
                                                        Linda Crofts

ACKNOWLEDGEMENTS

The editors would like to thank the following who kindly contributed their experiences as researchers to this book:

Allison Bell BSc RGN ENB100
Clinical Nurse Specialist – Pain Management, Royal Free Hospital, London, UK

C. Patricia Fathers MSc DipCNE(Edin) CertEd RGN OND(Hons) RM RNT
Senior Lecturer, School of Health, Biological and Environmental Sciences, Middlesex University, London, UK

Alison Hill RCN MSc Dip HV
Lead Nurse, Norfolk Cancer Network, UK

Anthony Pryce BA MSc PhD RGN RMN PGCEA RNT
DipSocPolRes
Director of Research, City University, London, UK

Common Research Items

The following glossary contains some common research items to aid the reader in critical analysis of research articles. For more detailed terms and definitions, *A Dictionary of Nursing Theory and Research* by B.A. Powers and T.R. Knapp (Sage Publications, 1990) makes an invaluable reference book for a department or ward. Reproduced by permission of Sage Publications.

Bias	Researchers are said to be biased if they are not objective when pursuing their research. A test is said to be biased if it is unduly difficult for one or more segments of some population.
Case study	A case study is an intensive, in-depth investigation of a single subject or a single unit, which could be a small number of individuals who seem to be representative of a larger group or very different from it.
Chi-square test	A test of statistical significance usually carried out on cross-tabulated data that summarise the relationship between two nominal variables.
Coding	Coding is a process of breaking down raw research data into some form in which they can be manipulated, organised and examined more easily.
Control group	In an experiment the control group is the group that does not receive the 'treatment' that is of particular interest to the researcher.
Delphi technique	The Delphi technique is a method for obtaining expert opinion on a topic, such as priorities in nursing research. It employs multiple 'rounds' or 'waves' of questionnaires with each round utilising information

gathered during previous rounds in an attempt to converge toward group consensus.

Dependent variable	The dependent variable in a research study is the variable that is of principal interest to the investigator, that is, the variable that really 'counts'.
Epistemology	Epistemology is a concept in philosophy that relates to theories of knowledge or how people came to have knowledge of the world.
Ethnography	Ethnography is a qualitative research approach developed by anthropologists. It is both a process and a product, the purpose of which is to describe a culture or particular aspect of a culture.
Experiment	An experiment is a study that involves manipulation of the principal independent variable, that is the actual administration of treatments or interventions that comprise the categories of the independent variable. An investigation is made of the effect of the independent variable on the dependent variable, e.g. the effect of Ventolin on asthma.
Fieldwork	A term borrowed from anthropology that is often used to describe the data-collection phase in qualitative research.
Grounded theory	A qualitative research approach developed by Glaser and Strauss in 1967 where the theory is 'grounded' in the data, i.e. the subjects being studied.
Hypothesis	A hypothesis is a statement that postulates some sort of relationship between concepts or between variables, e.g. patients who receive pre-operative information make a better recovery than those who receive no information.
Methodology	The design of the study and the actual procedures carried out in the collection and analysis of the data.
Phenomenology	A way of thinking about what life experiences are like for people – examines the world of human consciousness and perception.
Qualitative research	A cover term for a variety of research traditions originating in philosophy, anthropology, psychology and

	sociology. It is concerned with how people come to know the world in which they live.
Quantitative research	A cover term for empirical research traditions of the traditional sciences concerned with precise measurement, replicability, prediction and control. It includes techniques and procedures such as standardised tests, random sampling and tests of statistical significance.
Reliability	An instrument is reliable if it *consistently* measures what it is designed to measure.
Research	Research is a systematic process of investigation, the general purpose of which is to contribute to the body of knowledge that shapes and guides academic and/or practice disciplines.
Sampling	Sampling is the process of selecting a subset of objects from a larger set of objects, e.g. a sample of 200 nurses from a workforce of 2000.
Triangulation	Triangulation of data is used in qualitative studies as a way of confirming new information as it occurs over the course of data collection. Triangulation is the combined use of two or more theories, methods, data sources, investigators, or analysis methods in the study of the same phenomenon. To be considered triangulation the data must all have the same foci. The intent is to obtain diverse views of the phenomenon under study for purposes of validation.
Validity	An instrument is valid if it *accurately* measures what it is designed to measure.

How to Use this Book

Each chapter encompasses both qualitative and quantitative methodologies as the practicalities of conducting research are very similar, whichever approach you use. To help you find your way around the various sections we have used icons within the text to illustrate the main points.

Introductory points

These are found at the beginning of each chapter and summarise the chapter contents.

Time bombs

These are found within the body of the text and highlight particular issues that it is essential to address; otherwise these have a habit of 'exploding' later on and causing major problems.

Diaries

We have included diary extracts from active researchers. We hope these comments give a flavour of the experience of doing research.

Key points

These lists summarise the essential points to remember when planning and conducting your research.

Pitfall sections

These identify the most common problems that occur during the research process and give suggestions on how to prevent them as well as possible solutions if they should occur.

|

GETTING STARTED

Linda Crofts

- Choosing a topic
- Being realistic
- Resources
- Supervision and support

INTRODUCTION

There is little doubt that reading a chapter about getting started with your research is much easier than actually doing it. The purpose behind this chapter is to help you actually get going with your research rather than just vaguely thinking about it. There are essentially two types of individuals: the 'get well ahead' group and the avoiders. It is unlikely you have got this far in your academic life without knowing which group you belong to. Those of you in the former group probably do not need this chapter at all. You cannot bear leaving things to the last minute and have always done first drafts of assignments well ahead of the deadline just in case something happens to hold you up, like the children all getting chickenpox. For you, the pressure is in the doing of the assignment, not in managing the time.

If you are in the latter category then this chapter is for you. This group do an awful lot of thinking and reading and pondering before actually putting pen to paper and also find lots of other things to do on the day of writing, such as phoning friends and sorting out a bag of clothes for Oxfam. The first draft is usually the final draft with a bit of editing and it is usually produced fairly near the deadline. This group simply cannot work without the pressure of deadlines. (However, this group have always done their groundwork. They are quite different to those who dash off an essay the night before without any preparation who may well have come unstuck by now.) If this is you, then read on because you are going to find it very difficult to manage your research time effectively.

CHOOSING A TOPIC

Many textbooks will tell you that if you are doing research for the first time then you need to choose a topic that really grips you since you are going to be living and breathing the subject for a year plus. This is never as simple as it sounds. It is often the case that what you wish to research and what is researchable are two different things. If you are undertaking research as part of an academic award you may see this as an opportunity to address a question which has vexed you for much of your professional life, such as Why do health professionals still fail to manage pain adequately? or What are women most afraid of when being treated for breast cancer? In reality you are likely to have to narrow the focus of your topic down to a very specific aspect if you are going to keep within your word limit. If you are undertaking research because you wish to address a problem in practice you have the problem of striking a balance between doing a credible piece of work which is of relevance to nursing practice generally and still addressing your own particular local issue. If you are undertaking a piece of funded research then you may have been recruited to the project long after the research design has been established and therefore you have little say in the topic.

Whatever your chosen topic, there are several vital elements to consider when turning your idea into something researchable:

 What do you actually want to find out (in other words, what is the question?)?

 How much time have you got?

✔ Do you have a word limit?

✔ What resources are available to you?

What do you actually want to find out?

Few first-time researchers have a clear research question or hypothesis at the outset. It is more likely that you have an idea, topic or problem which you want to explore. At this initial stage of your research there is likely to be a lot of expanding and contracting of ideas and at this stage you want to expand the topic as much as possible so you can then tease out possible research questions. There are a couple of methods you can use to help you do this. First you can brainstorm your ideas onto a wall chart where you can see how your additions connect with earlier entries. More complex but very effective is a Mind Map or spidergram, as described by Tony Buzan (1989), with which lateral thinkers may already be familiar. This process of getting from topic to question can be demonstrated by the Mind Map shown in Figure 1.1, which illustrates discharge planning from hospital and the concern that it is not being carried out effectively.

This initial stage may well take a few weeks and you will need constant feeds of inspiration to keep adding to it. Inspiration can come from a number of sources; you may begin to do a bit of preliminary reading even if only that a current article catches your eye, but your best source is other people. Start talking to friends and colleagues about your interest and you will certainly begin to build

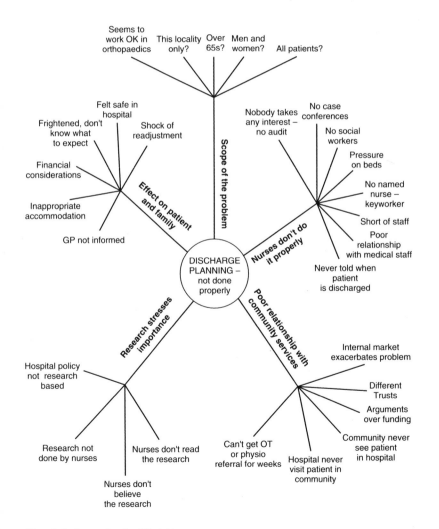

Fig. 1.1 *Example of a Mind Map*

up more ideas and gather different points of view. (As your work colleagues are likely to be used as sounding boards and props throughout your entire research project they may as well get used to talking about it now!) At this stage hoard everything and discard nothing.

'When I was near to starting my MSc research year I still didn't actually know what I was going to do; a colleague suggested looking at the perception of parents accompanying their children to theatre for an operation, which I rejected because I had very little clinical experience of caring for children. However, it got me thinking about why it was only children who were accompanied and my research eventually ended up about the involvement of relatives in acute adult care.'

Linda Crofts

From the Mind Map illustrated in Figure 1.1 it can be seen that already there are five clear avenues from the topic of discharge planning, any one of which has potential to provide a research question. You now want to test out possibilities by narrowing the field down. This is where you need to consider the time available to you, the word limit and the resources. If you have never done a research project before, how do you know what is actually achievable? The best person to advise you is your supervisor (which is discussed later in this chapter) but as a guide it is worth noting that Todd, Robinson and Reid took three years, full time, fully funded, to carry out their study of shift patterns in two hospitals in Northern Ireland. While it is true they studied the topic from a number of different angles and wrote numerous articles (Todd *et al.*, 1991, 1993; Reid *et al.*, 1993, 1994) the case remains that many of you are doing research projects part time in one year with a word limit of between 10 000 and 20 000 words. What you can realistically achieve is likely to be far less than what you would actually like to research (see Box 1.1).

In the example shown in Figure 1.1 we have seen that the topic of discharge planning breaks down into several distinct areas which, depending on the scope of your project, can either be studied individually, in a combination or, most likely, broken down even further. Box 1.2 shows some of the possibilities.

If you are well read on this topic you can probably add to the scope of this discussion as this example is by no means exhaustive.

Box 1.1 *What does 20 000 words look like?*

The best way to gauge what a BSc or MSc (or PhD) thesis looks like is to look at some. Colleagues may be happy to let you see their previous work and most university libraries keep copies of completed theses. A tutor once summarised the scope of the whole exercise by describing a 20 000 word thesis as 'eight assignments'. This was very helpful as the college guidelines for a thesis divided neatly into eight parts and some of the earlier assignments had been 2500 words. So, for a 10 000 word BSc project, imagine that your chapter on data collection is approximately 2000 words and you will see that it is actually *less* than some of your assignments. This may indicate that in our example of discharge planning you will have more than enough material by simply researching nursing practice on two hospital wards (maybe one good, one poor, or one male, one female, or whatever) while making only passing reference to the patient and family perspective, the scope of the problem and the relationship with community services. However with 20 000 words you may be able to incorporate one of these other aspects in the design.

Box 1.2 *Possible research areas in relation to the topic of discharge planning*

- Why are health professionals not taking notice of all the research that points towards the importance of good discharge planning for rehabilitation?
  (Is it doctors and nurses? Are they actually aware of the research? Do they believe it?)
- What is the scope of the problem?
  (Although it is a national issue are there areas where it is particularly problematic? Are there examples of good practice? Is it just elderly care?)
- What is the perspective of patients and carers?
  (What is their experience of discharge planning? Were they aware they had a discharge plan? Did anyone discuss it with them? What was the reality of follow-up in the community? How did their partners cope?)
- Is there a need to review nursing practice in relation to discharge planning and the factors that influence it?
  (Is it a unidisciplinary or multidisciplinary problem?)

Furthermore, if you are confident about doing action research, and you have someone to supervise you and your hospital has just drawn up a new policy you could do a study evaluating the implementation process of getting the policy into practice. The possibilities are endless.

In theory, it is once you have decided on your question/hypothesis that you then select your methodology and design your project. So, for example, the experience of patients and families would lend itself to a qualitative approach with some in-depth interviews as one of the main methods, whereas the relationship between hospital and community could be approached either as an experimental design with a null hypothesis (the relationship has no effect on the quality of discharge planning) or within a sociological framework to support a broadly descriptive study of the existing arrangements. In practice, novice researchers will often use a method they feel comfortable with (which may well be the method they described for their assignment in their research methods module) to fit the topic. If this is you then the initial exploratory phase of brainstorming/Mind Maps is even more important if you are to locate the range of possibilities that may benefit from the approach you most favour.

Many novice researchers are concerned that by limiting their study the assessor will not recognise that they have indeed considered the vast scope of their topic, but providing the limitations of the study (i.e. what it will and will not focus on) are spelt out in your terms of reference then there should be no problem in doing this. As an example, a nurse from the intensive therapy unit (ITU) sought advice on his BSc project. He was keen to do a study about stress in ITU staff and in particular whether the shift system was one of the contributory factors. He wanted to know if this had a negative effect on the quality of patient care. Not only did his study need to be far more specific in its focus but his word limit was 6000 words. On a topic as vast as stress he was unlikely to get much beyond the literature review before his word limit was up, let alone touch on any of the other topic areas.

On that point it is worth noting that a number of academic institutions have abandoned the final year research project for BSc students and instead ask for an extended literature review. This move is to be applauded. For some considerable time nursing has been guilty of conducting small-scale, ungeneralisable research when a thorough examination of the literature may well negate the need for the study altogether; nowhere is this more true than in the field of infection control. We do not need any more small-scale studies on hand washing, whereas a thorough review of the literature would inform and enlighten many a hospital policy and audit tool. As already highlighted above, it is also very difficult to produce a meaningful piece of research in 10 000 words, but you can do a very good literature review.

Those who insist that the only way of instilling the research process into students is to make them do it are missing the point; conducting an effective literature review and applying it to practice is surely what 'research-based practice' means.

What can you realistically achieve in a year?

Unless you are registered for a PhD, most of you will have approximately one year part-time to conduct your research. The purpose of narrowing your topic into something researchable (i.e. a specific question to ask or a hypothesis to test) is not purely to meet your word limit requirements but because the time you have to spend on this project is very restricted.

Those of you who are working as full-time researchers on one aspect of a big project will have different considerations, as the phasing of the project may already be determined and you are likely to be working as part of a team. If you are undertaking a piece of research unfunded and unsupported (i.e. you wish to explore a problem in practice just because it interests you), then your time will be even more limited unless your employer grants you time off to do the study. It has to be said that doing research in your spare time just for the love of it with no resources rarely comes to fruition. Research is hard work, time-consuming and can be lonely and without the carrot of an academic award or a paid research post you may well wonder why you bothered to start it. However, if this is you, then turn straight to the chapter on 'funding' as you may find that, having done the initial proposal, there are funds available to support the project which could pay for your release time out to do the study.

Managing time is a component of every management course yet few of us ever get it right. When it comes to your research project everyone will tell you how the time runs away with you, how everything takes twice as long as you planned and yet still, for many of you in October, the deadline of next September seems light years away. Surely it is far too early to start thinking about it now? The experience of those before you should tell you it is imperative to get started and certainly the advice of 'Think of it like eight assignments' helped get me going. One excellent tool to help you manage your time is the Gantt chart. These are primarily used in project management, a process that had its origins in the NASA space programme in the 1960s and has since been widely used in the construction industry and more recently in health care. Gantt charts are a more scientific, grown-up version of the fabulous revision timetables you drew up for yourself approaching your main school exams. Named after Henry Gantt, the industrial engineer who introduced the procedure in the early 1900s, a Gantt chart consists of a horizontal bar chart that graphically displays the time relationship of the steps of the project. Each step of a project is represented by a line placed on the chart in the time period when it is to be undertaken. When completed, the Gantt chart shows the flow of activities in sequence as well as those that can be underway at the same time. Figure 1.2 shows an example of how a Gantt chart might look for a one-year part-time research project.

'One of my concerns whilst conducting my research was to keep track of myself, my commitments, and my planned contact with my supervisor. I seemed to be writing and rewriting copious lists and using a series of adhesive notes stuck in my diary pages, which inevitably fell out as the glue faded. Then I remembered the Gantt charts I'd used while undertaking a project management job. I threw out the lists and sticker notes. Everything I needed to make a note of, deadlines both earliest and latest, my holidays! supervisor appointments, field days, stages of the work could all be seen on one page at a glance. It kept me sane and I felt in control of my time management.'

Patricia Fathers

An important aspect of a Gantt chart is that it does not only record your research work; other areas of your life are also included. Many nurses doing research have huge responsibilities at work, so if you know that April is always very busy you can plan to give minimal attention to your research that month. It is also unrealistic to expect that within the year you will not want to go away on holiday and that either you, your partner or your children will not be ill. You may even be expecting to move house (not to be recommended). Some, if not all of these events can be planned into your Gantt chart. For large-scale research projects, Gantt charts can be used as the basis for a detailed project plan, as is described in more detail in Chapter 7.

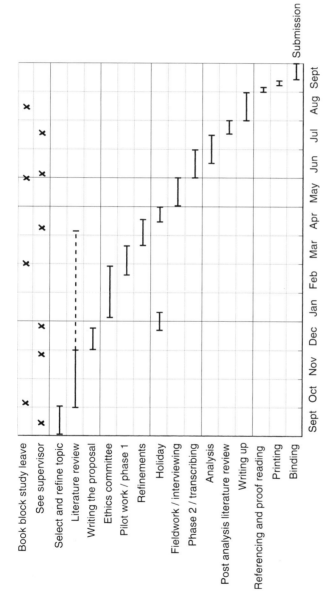

Fig. 1.2 *Example of a Gantt chart*

Resources, resources

Time is your most important resource and really the rest of this book is dedicated to helping you to make the most of it. However, there are a number of other resources you will need to undertake your research. These are:

- ✔ Libraries and source books
- ✔ Information technology
- ✔ A place to work
- ✔ Data collection tools
- ✔ Printing and binding facilities
- ✔ Academic supervision
- ✔ Moral support.

Libraries and source books

Using libraries effectively is described in detail in Chapter 3. However, there will come a time when it is clear that you will need to invest in some source books, i.e. textbooks on research describing different approaches to research. For many first-time researchers the problem is to determine which sources are reliable, particularly because many seem to be saying slightly different things or even contradict each other. Over time, however, you are likely to find yourself returning to one major text over and over again and providing it is reputable, this is the one to buy and stick to. In research terms alone, you are likely to need at least three textbooks: one academic research text, one that applies the theory to practice and a 'how to do it' book such as this volume. So, for example, Miles and Huberman (1994) gives you the definitive work on qualitative research but Silverman (2001) gives guidance on how to go about applying this to practice. In addition, you may want to seek out books which address the issues of research in your field; for example, Polgar and Thomas (2000) *Introduction to Research in the Health Sciences* sets research methods in the context of health care.

'Buy one good research textbook and use it for your basic information. Many of the books contradict each other so using just one book will help to ease this. You can always read more specialist books as the need arises or to clarify certain points.'

Alison Hill

Information technology

Extensive reference is made to utilising information technology (IT) in Chapters 3 and 7 in terms of using IT to access information sources. However, for many researchers either owning or having access to a personal computer which at least has word processing and spreadsheet facilities as well as the ability to produce simple statistics is seen as essential rather than an option. In theory, there is no reason why you cannot do all your drafts in long-hand and give the final draft to a skilled typist to produce the finished document. However, this can be very time-consuming in terms of proof-reading and sending it back and forth for amendments as well as bearing a financial cost. The majority of post-registration students use a word processor to produce their assignments and some academic institutions will no longer accept handwritten work.

There are considerable advantages to using a personal computer during your research project. It is easy to make amendments, 'cut and paste' and keep material apart in separate files. If you do not own your own computer then you almost certainly have access to one. All academic institutions have computers for student use, although there may not be many of them and demand for access can be high. However, your place of work may also have a computer you can use and it is worth asking around early on. If your hospital has a training and development centre and teaches computer skills you may be able to use the computers when they are not in use for training. Ask around and ensure you maximise your time when you are on the computer. If possible, avoid working with very old software simply because it is very slow and less likely to be compatible with other computers.

Make sure you save all your work on floppy disk, back it up and print out hard copies regularly. Never send your disk to anyone without having it copied first. It is advisable to spread your work over several disks in case of disasters. Rather like the principle of not keeping your cheque book and cheque card together, do not keep your disks and hard copies together either. Your research work is irreplaceable so treat it with respect.

A place to work

There will come a time in your research project when you need to take over a whole room. This is usually during the data analysis phase when you have data in neat piles everywhere, essential books to tell you how to do it, earlier chapters of your work printed out so you can cross-reference your analysis and so the list goes on. For qualitative studies this is a big issue as you may have multiple copies of interview transcripts in various stages of coding and 'cut and paste'.

Ideally, at this stage you should find yourself a room that can be devoted solely to your project for a period of time. Unless you live or work alone you will need to plan and negotiate this with either work colleagues or the people you live with. Perhaps a dining room or spare bedroom can be taken over for a couple of months? If you are using a Gantt chart or project plan you can at least roughly predict when this will be and give adequate warning. It can be particularly difficult to find such a space in a family home, but if your family have agreed to you taking over a room for a while then consider fitting a lock to it. These measures may sound extreme to first-time researchers, but in the crucial later stages you need the confidence to know that everything is exactly where you left it and that there is no danger that papers will be moved or lost.

Data collection tools

Before you start it is worth giving some consideration to the equipment you will need to conduct your research. If you are planning to tape record interviews make sure you know exactly how the tape recorder works. There are some neat little battery-operated recording machines available for under £40 if your budget can run to one; otherwise you have to resort to a standard radio/cassette player which is cumbersome and obtrusive. If you are asking participants to keep a reflective diary then you need to provide notebooks for them.

If you are using questionnaires then you need either to purchase them from the originator if they are published, validated tools (to avoid being in breach of copyright) or to have access to photocopying facilities if you are sending out multiple copies of your own questionnaire. This is covered in more detail in Chapter 9.

Printing and binding facilities

Many academic institutions insist on research projects being submitted bound in a hard jacket in the university colours. The easiest way to find out about binding facilities, if the information is not provided in your student handbook, is to ask last year's students. Well-established universities often have an arrangement with a binder who knows exactly what the university regulations are and even the submission dates. Newer institutions do not. You therefore need to consult your local Yellow Pages to find out if there is a binder near you who can do academic work. You will of course need to spell out in detail the exact university requirements.

Do make sure you leave enough time at the end for this, most binders need at least a fortnight clear. Binding is also expensive and you will have to foot the bill for this yourself.

'I used a local binder, recommended by a colleague who had used them the year before and they had told me simply to ring when I was ready and they would make sure it was done in time. I was a week late because there had been problems with printing and when I phoned, the receptionist told me they were closed for three weeks as they were moving premises. I thought my whole world was about to collapse but in the end the registry agreed to take soft bound copies in lieu of the real thing.'

Linda Crofts

If you have produced all your work on disk but do not have access to a high-quality printer this can also be problematic. By far the cheapest option is to ask a family member, friend or colleague who does have access to such facilities to do it for you. If you have to resort to an outside company then it is going to be expensive. Your disk is unlikely to format exactly so small adjustments have to be made; for example, your columns may need realignment. Computer time is £60 per hour upwards and the printing costs are on top of this. These days you can purchase inkjet and laser printers for under £200 and this may be worth considering if you are about to resort to a commercial printing company.

Academic supervision

The arrangements for academic supervision vary from one academic institution to another; some allocate two supervisors and expect you to use both, others allocate one and expect you to work pretty much on your own. Your guidance notes will tell you the maximum time you can have with your academic supervisor unless there are real problems.

The relationship between academic supervisor and supervisee is very much a two-way process. The best supervisor in the world can do nothing for a student who demands to meet at extremely short notice, cancels appointments or does not turn up and has nothing prepared when the meeting does take place. Equally, students get extremely frustrated with supervisors who can never be contacted, hang on to their work for months, then forget they have it and appear to have little or no interest in the students or their work. It is the bane of every student's research year to find that when they need their supervisor most (i.e. over the summer) they are away on sabbatical for three months and did not think to let the student know.

So what are the features of a constructive relationship? Essentially supervisor and supervisee must have confidence in each other and respect each other's point of view. The relationship should have the features of a good learning contract, i.e. recognise that each other's time is valuable. Every attempt should be made to keep appointments unless cancellation is unavoidable and to ensure that the appointment is fruitful. Students should produce draft chapters on time and supervisors should give feedback promptly.

It is not the supervisor's job to tell the student what to do but rather discuss options and equally the students should not expect supervisors to do the research for them. However, supervisors are in a position to advise on whether the work conforms to university standards and guidelines, and that the student is on the right track, and students should heed this advice.

'I was fortunate to have a very good supervisor. She was available on the phone at home if needed. Even allowing for this it was still sometimes difficult to arrange a mutually convenient time, particularly over university holidays. In total I had only about eight supervisions (MSc) over six months; however, each was longer than an hour and I came away with plenty to think about.'

Alison Hill

Some institutions ask students to submit an outline proposal at the beginning of their research year so that appropriate supervisors can be allocated. This can be difficult as the original idea may bear no resemblance to the fully worked-up proposal several months later. Ideally you will be allocated two supervisors, one whose expertise is in your research methodology and the other whose expertise is in your topic area. In practice this is rarely the case, partly because your plan may alter quite radically but mostly because your ideal supervisor may already be over-committed, or indeed, simply not exist. If you are able to choose your supervisor and the institution only allows one, then as a first-time researcher you are probably best advised to choose someone whose expertise is in the methodology you have selected rather than the topic. It is your ability to understand and apply the research process that will ultimately determine whether you pass or not, regardless of how well you know your subject.

It is important to admit when supervision is not working. If you lack confidence in your supervisor or feel that he or she lacks confidence in you and you feel you are getting nowhere, then make an appointment to see your Director of Studies. Changing supervisors halfway through can be very disruptive to your work so make quite sure that you consider what you could do yourself to improve the situation before you decide to change supervisor.

Moral support

'During my BSc dissertation I could only talk about two things, my research and the soaps on TV. One was a distraction from the other and it was as though nothing else existed in my life.'

Alison Bentley

Research can be a very lonely business. If a topic really grabs you and some fascinating revelations come out of the fieldwork you become totally absorbed in your research to the exclusion of everything else. What can be so disappointing is that nobody else really seems to know what you are talking about and you notice a slightly impatient twitch on the face of your loved ones as you embark on your story of what you found out today. There are also moments of deep depression when your data do not fit, you feel way out of your depth and writer's block has set in.

It is very important to have a network around you of people you can talk to about your research. Your academic supervisor is obviously very important but should not be your sole source of support. It may be that there is a research support group at your college where lecturers and students alike can discuss research problems informally and share ideas. Some large hospitals may also have this. It can be very reassuring to find you are not the only one who feels a bit at sea.

If your organisation has a senior nurse responsible for research then make contact with him or her. This nurse almost certainly knows of other nurses also doing research that you could meet up with, may well hold informal sessions and can offer invaluable advice when you come to the fieldwork stage in terms of 'opening doors' into areas you want to use for your research.

Talk to colleagues who have done research in the past. They will remember what it was like and can offer tips as well as comfort and support.

> 'During the year I undertook my MSc research I shared my office with a colleague who was also a friend in the institution where we both worked as nurse teachers. Not only did she have invaluable advice about keeping on track as well as lending me books and other resources but she also shouldered a considerable proportion of my teaching load for the last few months so I could free myself up to finish my research. I realise that not everyone is as lucky as this but finding an informal mentor in someone who did their research last year can be invaluable.'
>
> Linda Crofts

Above all, keep a sense of humour. When you are totally immersed in your research and things start to go wrong it is easy to get things out of perspective. You are almost certainly not much fun to live with, so try to keep some semblance of a social life, go away for the odd long weekend and do try to see the funny side when the patient you go to interview does not speak English, the patient is not in hospital any more, the patient declines consent at the last minute.... It is all part of doing research; it is not the end of the world.

KEY POINTS

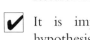

- There is a world of difference between the topic you want to research and what is researchable.

- It is imperative to have a clear research question or hypothesis.

- Mind Maps and Gantt charts are useful aids for helping to define the scope of your research and plan your time.

- Be realistic about what is achievable within your word limit and time-frame.

- Invest in essential textbooks and some basic information technology.

Having somewhere to work is essential and having people around you can talk to makes the research process far more manageable.

 Academic supervisors and supervisees have a responsibility towards each other and should respect each other's views.

COMMON PITFALLS AND HOW TO AVOID THEM

Pitfall	Solution
The topic is too broad	Use a Mind Map to plot the scope and dimensions of your topic then be prepared to narrow the focus down to one specific aspect.
Vague research question	Define what it is you actually want to find out. Set aims and objectives. Then formulate a very clear research question or draw up a testable hypothesis.
Inability to visualise size of the thesis	Break down the word limit into manageable chunks by imagining the chapters are sequential assignments. Look at previous researchers' work.
Inability to manage the long period of time, keep thinking you have 'loads of time to spare'	Draw up a Gantt chart and stick to it to demonstrate to yourself you do not have time to spare, indeed the opposite is true. Remember to plan for holidays and printing/binding time at the end.
The research textbooks all seem to contradict each other	Choose one reputable textbook which you find readable and stick to it.
Do not have own personal computer	You almost certainly have access to one. Ask student services at your university and ask around your hospital or place of work.

Your draft chapters have gone missing in the post	Make regular copies of all your work and keep your PC disks separate from hard copies. Spread your work over several disks for insurance.
Supervisor always unavailable and does not seem to know what your research is about	Make sure you do your utmost to keep contact with your supervisor and do not break appointments unnecessarily. Have something prepared to discuss. If your efforts are in vain consider changing supervisor.
You feel totally isolated and depressed because no-one seems to understand what you are going through	Keep a sense of humour. Make contact with fellow researchers and make use of research support sessions. Try not to make the lives of your nearest and dearest unbearable.

REFERENCES

Buzan, T. (1989) *Use Your Head*. London: BBC Books.

Miles, M.B. and Huberman, A.M. (1994) *Qualitative Data Analysis: An expanded sourcebook*, 2nd edition. Thousand Oaks, CA: Sage.

Polgar, S. and Thomas, S.A. (2000) *Introduction to Research in the Health Sciences*, 4th edition. Melbourne: Churchill Livingstone.

Reid, N., Robinson, G. and Todd, C. (1993) The quantity of nursing care on wards working 8- and 12-hour shifts. *International Journal of Nursing Studies* **30**(5): 403–413.

Reid, N., Robinson, G. and Todd, C. (1994) The twelve hour shift: the views of nurse educators and students. *Journal of Advanced Nursing* **19**: 938–946.

Silverman, D. (2001) *Interpreting Qualitative Data*, 2nd edition. Thousand Oaks, CA: Sage.

Todd, C., Reid, N. and Robinson, G. (1991) The impact of 12-hour nursing shifts. *Nursing Times* **87**(31): 47–50.

Todd, C., Robinson, G. and Reid, N. (1993) 12-hour shifts: Job satisfaction of nurses. *Journal of Nursing Management* **1**: 215–220.

2

THE CONTEXT OF RESEARCH IN THE NHS

Linda Crofts

- Clinical effectiveness
- Clinical governance
- Evidence-based practice
- Practice development
- Research and development

INTRODUCTION

Before going any further with your project it is important to have some understanding of the context of research in the NHS. There are a number of reasons why even the first-time novice researcher needs to be aware of what the concepts listed above mean in practice. Most of these terms were almost unheard of prior to 1995 but since then have significantly impacted on many health care professionals' ability to access research findings, critique research and use research findings in practice. Apart from gaining an understanding of these concepts to help inform everyday practice, it is also essential that before embarking on any research project you are able to assess accurately how your research may contribute to the existing evidence and how it is likely to impact on practice.

CLINICAL EFFECTIVENESS

Clinical effectiveness is doing the right thing in the right way and at the right time for the right patient (Royal College of Nursing, 1996). Many nurses equate this with the 'five Rs' many learnt as student nurses when learning how to give a drug safely (right patient, right drug, right dose, right route, right time) and indeed one could argue that safe administration of medication is effective practice, providing that we are confident that 'the extent to which specific clinical interventions, when deployed in the field for a particular patient or population, do what they are intended to do, that is, maintain and improve health and secure the greatest possible health gain from the available resources' (NHS Executive, 1996).

For many health care professionals, the concept of clinical effectiveness is problematic in terms of its very existence. Why do we need a term called clinical effectiveness when no health care professional would ever like to think they give care and treatment that is ineffective? The answer is that we may think the care we give is effective but we do not always know that this is actually the case. Research takes time to publish and appear in journals, busy health care professionals do not always have time to read the latest research or may not know how to read it and in any case, are unlikely to be able to access the huge range of material on the topic. What has been increasingly shown is that most practitioners practice from a knowledge base that is built up through experience but is not necessarily questioned or updated.

Treatment and care costs are rising all the time and any government needs to feel confident that the public purse is paying for treatment and care that is effective and not those treatments that have no known benefit. While this was the clear message behind the Executive framework laid out in 1996, many practitioners know that treatment and care cannot simply be divided into those interventions that are effective and those that are not. Many of our current practices lie somewhere in the middle for the following reasons:

- There may not yet be enough research that overwhelmingly endorses a treatment yet patients seem to benefit from it and there are no other effective alternatives (some cancer treatments fall in this category).
- Not all treatments can be assessed through conventional drug or intervention trials. Many complementary therapies fall into this category. Critics say there is not enough evidence of their effectiveness in the form of drug trials; advocates say that complementary therapies are frequently part of a holistic approach to well-being and cannot be tested in such a reductionist way. The same arguments prevail over such therapies as counselling; some GP practices fund counselling, others do not on the grounds it is difficult to prove its effectiveness.
- Effectiveness studies are usually about a single disease base (e.g. asthma) yet human beings often present to their doctors with a

multitude of interwoven problems which just do not fit into neat categories.

- Many nursing interventions are around health education, inter-personal care and patient support, often grouped under the heading 'the Art of Nursing'. Again, this is notoriously difficult to quantify.
- Today's absolute truth is tomorrow's history. While we practise today from a secure knowledge base, tomorrow we discover a break-through that questions everything we thought to be true. There are examples across health care too numerous to mention, but simply in the area of tissue viability, many of the current guidelines for good practice would have had a previous generation of nurses reeling; many wound care products used in my training days are now known to be detrimental to the healing process and even the humble sheep-skin is now known to hinder the healing of pressure sores rather than help prevent them.

While recognising that we cannot always be sure that the treatment and care we give is scientifically proven to be effective, never-theless it is important that all practitioners question their practice and strive to make it as effective as possible. Clinical effectiveness is an umbrella term for a range of different skills, tools and resources which hang together to create an all-embracing approach to quality improvement. As we can see from Figure 2.1, clinical effectiveness attempts to bring together clinical audit, clinical risk management, education and training, which highlights the need for practitioners

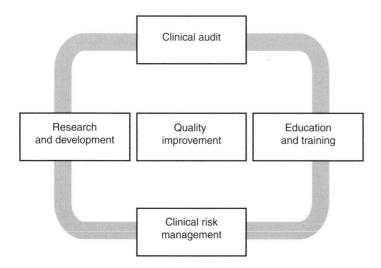

Fig. 2.1 *Clinical effectiveness*

to develop skills in accessing and appraising research and using this to develop protocols and research and development.

CLINICAL GOVERNANCE

While the literature abounds with definitions of clinical governance, in my view it may best be described as clinical effectiveness with teeth. The relationship between clinical effectiveness and clinical governance needs to be traced back to the end of the health care reforms at the end of the 1990s and the subsequent White Paper 'The New NHS; Modern. Dependable (1997) and its sister paper 'A First Class Service' (NHS Executive, 1998a). The NHS during the 1990s was characterised by the creation of the internal market in which it was believed that by introducing competition between health care providers care and treatment would be more efficient. Towards the end of the life of the internal market it was clear not only that health care was not more efficient, primarily due to the large duplication of services offered by competing providers and the cost of administrating complex cross-charging systems, but also that it was not particularly effective. The responsibility of the Chief Executive of an NHS Trust was to be corporately accountable for the financial position of the Trust and provided a Trust did not step outside existing legislation, the Trust Board was free to manage the Trust as they saw fit to do so. In many cases this meant that Trusts had to compete for contracts which were usually awarded on the basis of cost but not necessarily quality.

While providing a quality service within finite resources remains an intractable problem to the NHS, the internal market was particularly problematic to clinicians who were trying to provide an acceptable standard of care in a cost-driven environment. Those involved in the early days of clinical audit, quality circles or research and development were often demoralised by the growing awareness that there was little support from senior colleagues in terms of time or money to pursue such activities, as they were often seen as peripheral to the core business of remaining solvent. Thus the launch of the clinical effectiveness strategy (NHS Executive, 1996) unsurprisingly made little impact at the time.

The reforms of 1997 were, and are still, perhaps the most ambitious plans yet to modernise the NHS and meet the comprehensive health needs of the UK population. Amongst a whole raft of reforms that set out to replace the internal market was the concept of clinical governance defined as 'A Framework through which

NHS organisations are accountable for continuously improving the quality of their services and safeguarding high standards of care by creating an environment in which excellence in clinical care will flourish' (NHS Executive, 1998b).

This statement on first reading can appear quite innocuous, simply promoting the idea of providing quality care, until one focuses on the key word 'accountable'. Clinical governance now means that the Chief Executive of a Trust is not only responsible for the corporate position of the Trust but also the clinical standards of care and treatment.

Four years into the reforms, many Trusts remain in a constant whirlwind of activity around clinical governance from developing and implementing risk management strategies, reviewing systems for determining clinical incompetence, striving to meet standards from the National Service Frameworks and investing in education and training. It is suggested that to date this has simply resulted in complex Trust systems being developed and implemented so that information can be routinely presented to the Trust Board, with little discernible impact on organisational culture (Walshe et al., 2000). However, I would argue it has had an impact on the ability of nurses to get their voices heard when they wish to pursue quality improvements for their patients. There has been a significant amount of innovation over the last few years, particularly in the form of nurse-led initiatives such as assessment clinics, integrated care pathways and health education, all of which has been against a backdrop of increased workload. While it would be wrong to argue that innovation did not exist before the reforms – it clearly did, as the Nurse Development Units can testify – there is no doubt that it is now much easier to get support for initiatives that can demonstrate more efficient and effective ways to care for patients. It is therefore imperative that such initiatives can be systematically evaluated to ensure that their effectiveness can be measured.

EVIDENCE-BASED PRACTICE

The term 'evidence-based practice' has been derived from evidence-based medicine, a concept which became prevalent around the same time as clinical effectiveness. It was aimed at providing better research-based information to doctors, mostly in the form of guidelines and protocols to assist with clinical decision-making. However, it quickly became apparent that using the evidence is not just about clinical outcomes, it is also about resources and values (Muir-Gray, 1997). While it would be nice to think that this development came about because Whitehall genuinely wished patients to receive better care, it is alas the result of simple expediency. Ineffective health care costs more than effective health care and runs the added risk of doing the patient harm, thus costing Trusts dear in terms of litigation. It became clear that such a concept would have only limited impact if restricted to medicine and that to be truly clinically effective, principles of evidence-based practice needed to apply to all settings across the whole spectrum of multiprofessional working.

Before moving on to examine the various strengths and weaknesses of evidence-based practice, we need to identify what it actually is and its constituent parts. Sackett *et al.* (1997) describe it as 'Integrating individual clinical expertise with the best available external evidence from systematic research'. Thus we can see that evidence-based practice is much more than simply applying particular research findings. It is cumulative research, appraised and condensed systematically and used to support clinical expertise, not replace it.

The five types of evidence

For the purpose of conducting a meta-analysis or systematic review, the NHS Centre for Reviews and Dissemination (CRD) classify research into five categories (Box 2.1). CRD have been at pains to point out that such a classification does not suggest that quantitative, experimental research is better, or more highly rated than other types of research but alas, many health care professionals interpret the categories to mean just that in terms of evidence, thereby supporting the assumption that the randomised controlled trial is king. In particular, nursing feels it fares at a particular disadvantage; as a relative late-comer to research, nursing has been struggling to establish a research identity for itself distinctive from medicine by concentrating on research broadly in the qualitative paradigm. Such research would be classified in categories IV and V.

However, in terms of carrying out systematic reviews and meta-analysis of treatment interventions, it is not surprising that the most effective approach is to compare like with like, to which most experimental designs lend themselves very well. Qualitative research is more difficult to review systematically as it is often about the illness experience and rarely generalisable. In some cases where reviews have been attempted, the results have been disappointing; Hale *et al.* (1999) carried out a limited review of managed care, integrated care pathways and case management to identify the seeds of an evidence base and found that very few publications were actually properly designed research studies. However, at the other end of the continuum,

Box 2.1 *Classification of research by the NHS Centre for Reviews and Dissemination*

I Strong evidence from at least one published systematic review of multiple, well-designed randomised controlled trials.

II Strong evidence from at least one published properly designed randomised controlled trial of appropriate size and in an appropriate clinical setting.

III Evidence from published well-designed trials without randomisation, single group pre-post, cohort, time series or matched case-controlled studies.

IV Evidence from well-designed non-experimental studies from more than one centre or research group.

V Opinions of respected authorities, based on clinical evidence, descriptive studies or reports of expert consensus committees.

Alison Tierney, in her keynote address to the International Nursing Research conference in 1998 cited the review by Winningham *et al.* (1994), which confirms fatigue as the most frequently reported and troublesome symptom of cancer and its treatments for all ages in all groups and concludes that patients attribute loss of quality of life to fatigue. This systematic review of all types of research, including many qualitative studies, is clearly important in terms of informing nursing practice.

Whatever the shortcomings of such a classification system, these are early days in the evidence-based health care (EBHC) movement and no doubt many lessons will be learnt along the way. Nevertheless, EBHC is now woven into the fabric of the NHS modernisation agenda and therefore it is helpful to examine its strengths and weaknesses.

Strengths

EBHC may help providers to make better use of limited resources, thus reducing rationing

This role is increasingly being seen as a major part of the work of the National Institute of Clinical Excellence (NICE), which will be discussed later. One of the absolute givens in health care is that demand will always outstrip supply. It is also the case that although there is no explicit NHS agenda around rationing, the reality is very different.

The strengths of EBHC is that where clinicians and managers are trying to make decisions within finite resources, such decisions are better made on the basis of effectiveness rather than pure cost alone. For example, investing in pressure-relieving mats for use on hospital trolleys for vulnerable patients effectively reduces the incidence of pressure sores which are costly to both the hospital and the individual in terms of their treatment and well-being.

EBHC may improve continuity and uniformity of care

One of the problems we experience in health care is that practice can vary between one provider and another; for example, a patient experiencing a hospital admission for an asthma attack may receive different types of treatment in different hospitals which changes again in primary care. By using evidence to provide national guidance for specific disease-related groups, as NICE has done, patients should expect that they receive consistent, effective treatment wherever they happen to be.

EBHC enables clinicians to spend more time thinking through the implications with the individual

In the past, a tremendous amount of time in medical education focused on medical students cramming their heads full of endless medical facts, much of which they would never be called on to use. The human brain is not like a computer database but using the two together can be hugely beneficial. A clinician who is able to assess the scenario in front of him or her and then able to access electronically the latest evidence can spend more time talking about treatment options that best suit the patient and their lifestyle. This can be as simple as knowing that a child presenting with a chest infection which would benefit from antibiotics has a range of choices, such as clarithromycin or co-amoxiclav; both do a similar job but one is taken twice a day and one three times a day. For a working mother, opting for a treatment that is given twice a day saves her needing to involve the daytime carer in a midday dose, thus making it more likely that the course is administered effectively.

External clinical evidence may replace tradition and ritual within health care setting

One of the biggest challenges to the implementation of EBHC is to invite clinicians to question their practice, which they may be continuing simply out of habit. This is very difficult to achieve not least because 'you don't know what you don't know'. This is particularly difficult with preventative treatments, a prime example being childhood immunisations. In general, we believe immunisation to be effective in a mass population. However, critics claim that it is improvements in social living standards that are responsible for the eradication of some childhood diseases rather than immunisations and that the side effects of some immunisations mitigate against their widespread use. But how will we ever know? To stop doing something preventative is highly risky unless we have overwhelming evidence to the contrary. This aside, the challenge is to change a culture of reliance on self-knowledge to one where clinicians regularly consult EBHC databases and NICE and are open to questioning their practice.

EBHC assists in developing audits of quality associated with clinical governance

Because EBHC lends itself to the development of protocols and standards these can be audited. The clearest examples of these on a national scale are the National Service Frameworks, which are designed to ensure consistent standards of care (for example for cancer) across the NHS (and increasingly the private sector). This provides much greater opportunities not only for departments to audit themselves but also to compare themselves with other providers (comparative data sets), thus constantly seeking to improve on the status quo.

EBHC represents a common multidisciplinary language

The guidance issued by NICE and the National Service Frameworks are aimed at groups of patients not groups of staff. As all health care professionals are responsible for the implementation of such guidance it provides a real opportunity for the multidisciplinary team to work together around and with the patient rather than purely from a professional base. The benefits of multidisciplinary teamwork have long been advocated; it is quite another thing getting groups of staff in fairly entrenched positions to actually practise it.

Weaknesses

EBHC is concerned with efficiency and effectiveness and may deny other values in society

Because EBHC is disease-specific, critics argue that it mitigates against holistic care giving and that values other than efficiency and effectiveness may be ignored. For example, it has taken a long time for the new drug Aricept (donepezil), designed to slow the progression of Alzheimer's disease, to get approval from NICE. This has evoked criticism from some quarters that the reason for the delay was that the disease mainly affects the elderly and that elderly people are not valued in society. If EBHC is to be embraced by health professionals it needs to clearly state the relationship between clinical effectiveness and cost effectiveness.

Clinicians may see EBHC as a threat

Medical staff in particular have seen their power base in health care rapidly deteriorating in recent years and could be naturally suspicious of any initiative that could be seen to cause further erosion. It is important that EBHC and attendant clinical guidelines are seen as tools that support and assist clinical decision-making, not replace it. If a clinician does not feel a protocol is applicable to the patient in front of them for good clinical reasons then they need to feel they have scope for justifying alternative treatments in such cases.

There is a lack of tools for evaluating the impact of EBHC on clinical and managerial decisions

Evaluative research is increasingly making its long overdue entry into health care settings as means of identifying benefits and drawbacks to patients, carers, staff and organisations in a wide range of service developments. EBHC still needs to be implemented on a wider scale with easy access to EBHC databases before such evaluation can take place, during which time much of the current evidence may have changed.

May be one more change to add to an already overburdened NHS

It is important that EBHC is not seen simply as 'another thing to do' but as a resource underpinning clinical decision-making. For EBHC to be seen as an effective resource that assists rather than hinders clinicians, the poor beleaguered NHS information technology needs to be catapulted into the twenty-first century. Despite the setting up of the NHS Information Authority, who are charged with the delivery of the ambitious 'Information for Health' strategy (NHS Executive, 1998b), in reality information technology in the NHS is in poor shape, with many clinical areas in hospitals, health centres and clinics experiencing poor or non-existent access to computers, an over-emphasis on managerial information rather than clinical information and poor compatibility with the outside world. If clinicians are to apply EBHC to everyday practice they need easy, reliable access to electronic information.

Most effective treatments are not necessarily the cheapest

Increasingly, NICE have taken over the role of assessing clinical effectiveness and cost effectiveness of treatments and are clear that value for money should not be confused with cheapness. Memories of the internal market are still fresh in collective memories and many nurses could and did tell managers that buying cheaper dressing swabs just means you use more of them and is therefore not cost effective. On the other hand we know there are real savings to be had by using generic drugs rather than branded ones that are exactly the same. Cost effectiveness needs to be visible in improved patient outcomes if clinicians are to be convinced that effectiveness is not being compromised by cheapness.

EBHC will need to be incorporated into policy decisions

This is increasingly becoming apparent as the National Service Frameworks come into effect. Trusts will need to demonstrate how they are meeting the minimum standards set out in the Frameworks and therefore these are now well integrated into local policy.

We can therefore see that EBHC is far reaching but far from straightforward. However, as the last point clearly states, EBHC is increasingly woven into the fabric of everyday health care. The problem for the busy clinician is not always where to use EBHC but where to find it.

Sources of evidence

Not so very long ago, if you wanted to know more about a particular topic you faced a fairly lengthy, labour-intensive half day in the post-graduate or university library undertaking a literature review of your topic, hoping that your searching techniques were adequate to get you the information you needed. It is increasingly recognised that one of the main obstacles to the implementation of EBHC is time and resources. There are now increasing numbers of databases that health care professionals can access that have essentially done much of the searching, reviewing and critiquing for them. This sub-ject is described in more detail in Chapter 3, but the new National Electronic Library for Health (NELH) at this moment still under construction, will be considered the most definitive resource on cur-rent evidence available to all, both clinicians and any other Internet users. This raises the spectacle of twenty-first century health care comprising of clinician and patient both being able to access reliable information at the point of consultation; for the patient this is most likely to be in the form of a dedicated patient information sheet. The challenge for the NHS in fact is not in relation to EBHC, but an effective information technology strategy that means com-puter access for clinicians is essential. At present this is far from the case.

National Institute of Clinical Excellence

As well as the NELH, the National Institute for Clinical Excellence (NICE) is also now in place. NICE was set up as a Special Health Authority in 1998 and its role is to produce authoritative national guidance as part of an overall approach to achieving consistent clinical standards across the NHS. The rationale behind the establish-ment of NICE is that if there are clear, evidence-based national standards this will reduce variations in treatment and care. NICE has two main roles: to 'horizon scan' by identifying new interven-tions and products under development at an early stage in order to assess the potential significance for the NHS and to appraise and provide guidance on existing interventions. To this end NICE posts clinical guidance based on the available evidence on its website (www.nice.org.uk). Guidance ranges from fairly straightforward conditions such as asthma, diabetes and hip replacements through to the availability of NHS hearing aids and more controversial drugs, such as beta-interferon. NICE has brought together a number of dif-ferent agencies such as the National Prescribing Centre's Appraisals and Bulletins and the National Centre for Clinical Audit.

Linked closely to the work of NICE are the National Service Frameworks (NSFs), which can be found on the Department of Health's website at www.doh.gov.uk. Based on the available evi-dence, these lay down the minimum standards of treatment and care for specific disease groups such as cancer, coronary heart disease, mental health and elderly care. If you are considering doing any research around these four topics you should look carefully at these standards as it is quite possible that you will need to take account of these standards in your work. For example, if you were interested in how long women have to wait for a consultant referral for a suspected breast lump you will need to know that the national minimum standard is two weeks and therefore there is published clinical audit identifying how far hospitals are reaching this target. Increasingly local health care is based on national directives and it is important you make that your starting point when designing your research project.

Using evidence in practice

In order to use evidence to support practice there are some key skills all health care professionals need:

- Skills in literature searching, both in libraries and on-line
- Information technology skills
- Turning a literature search into a review
- Abilities in critiquing and appraising research studies
- Applying the findings to the development of locally based guide-lines and protocols.

As we can see, many of these skills are those needed to conduct a research project and are discussed in detail in subsequent chapters of this book. However, it is also my view that evidence-based practice, like many of its fellow NHS concepts, suffers from a perennial problem in that many journal articles assume everyone knows how to practice from an evidence base without addressing the overwhelming training and education need that will necessarily accompany its implementation. This is characterised by the fact that some five years after its introduction, training places on workshops remain as popular as ever. To really practise from an evidence base, health care professionals need a thorough grounding in research training and this has been very patchy up until now. One could cynically argue that nursing, in particular, being a relative newcomer to research has simply moved from 'Sister says ... ' to 'Research says ... ' to 'the evidence says ... ' while the knowledge based for practice has barely shifted. Within medicine O'Donnell (1997) offers an equally sceptical view, stating 'Clinical experience, which used to involve making the same mistakes with increasing confidence over an impressive number of years has been replaced by "evidence based medicine" which involves perpetuating other people's mistakes instead of your own.'

Cynicism apart, it is fair to say that clinical practice is as much to do with perceiving as it is knowing. As Naish (1997) says: 'Nursing is a messy area in which to introduce evidence based practice. You can't just slavishly apply evidence'. In the same article, Naish goes on to quote AM Rafferty who states:

> EBP has been cast as a simplistic solution but practitioners and policy makers must adopt a sophisticated view. EBP can make nurses responsible for issues that are beyond their control, unless they are in an environment such as a Nursing Development Unit where nurse led and evidence based cultures are adequately supported. EBP moves accountability down the line to practitioners and unless it is vested with real substantive power, then you are creating unrealistic expectations.

THE ROLE OF PRACTICE DEVELOPMENT

Salvage (1998) claims that 'While nursing may not have much research, we've got lots of documented developmental works, such as the NDU [Nursing Development Unit] movement, which puts nursing as a front runner in initiating change management.' While there is some truth in this statement, as we have already seen, in that nursing does not always lend itself easily to EBHC; it is also unfortunately, with some notable exceptions in relation to Nursing Development Units, the case that a lot of practice development has not been systematically evaluated in a way that would allow it to stand up to scrutiny. It may be that nurses engaged in practice development do not possess research skills that would allow them to identify the scope of an evaluative study, or it may be that it is perceived that practice development is 'easier' than research. Whatever the reasons, the result has been that much practice development has only been written up from an individual, anecdotal perspective, making it difficult to generalise. The result has been that much good practice development has failed to stand up to scrutiny, not because the idea was flawed but because of the lack of systematic evaluation.

Practice development is often the most relevant area for many health care professionals to research yet has often been overlooked. However, in NHS research and development terms, the new funding arrangements under 'Priorities and Needs' make clear that evaluation of services, organisation of care and practice development are a priority. For many nurses there could not be a clearer reason for equipping themselves with research skills so they are able to contribute to a much needed evidence base for practice.

CONCLUSION

The purpose of this chapter is to guide potential researchers through a critical first stage in the research process, which is to ask yourself 'Are you sure you need to do a research project?' So often the researcher's enthusiasm for the subject gets the better of them and it is easy to find yourself undertaking a project for which there is already sufficient evidence available. Research projects need to strengthen the evidence base, not duplicate them. Understanding and utilising evidence in practice is perhaps an even more critical skill than undertaking a project at all.

Finally, before starting your research project, ask yourself the following questions:

 Are you sure someone hasn't already done your project?

Are you making assumptions about what is already known about this topic?

How are you going to find out what evidence is already out there?

 Do you need to rethink the aim of your project in order to complement, not duplicate, available evidence?

Are there any published national standards you need to take into account?

In order to help you answer these questions, the next chapter will take you through how to undertake a literature search and review.

REFERENCES

Hale, C., Crofts, L. and Stokoe, L. (1999) Managed care, case management and multi-disciplinary pathways of care: a selective review for the RCN R&D priority-setting exercise. *NTResearch* **4**(5): 366–377.

Muir Gray, J.A. (1997) *Evidence-based Healthcare – How to Make Health Policy and Management Decisions.* Edinburgh: Churchill Livingstone.

Naish, J. (1997) So where's the evidence? *Nursing Times* **93**(12): 64–66.

NHS Executive (1996) *Promoting Clinical Effectiveness; a Framework for Action in and through the NHS.* London: HMSO.

NHS Executive (1997) *The New NHS; Modern. Dependable.* London: HMSO.

NHS Executive (1998a) *A First Class Service; Quality in the New NHS.* London: HMSO.

NHS Executive (1998b) *Information for Health.* London: HMSO.

O'Donnell, M. (1997) *A Sceptic's Medical Dictionary.* London: BMJ Publishing.

Royal College of Nursing (1996) *Clinical Effectiveness.* London: RCN.

Sackett, D.L., Richardson, W.S., Rosenberg, W. and Haynes, R.B. (1997) *Evidence-based Medicine; How to Practise and Teach Evidence-based Medicine*. Edinburgh: Churchill Livingstone.

Salvage, J. (1998) Evidence-based practice: a mixture of motives? *Nursing Times* **94**(23): 61–63.

Tierney, A. (1998) The leading edge in nursing research. *NTResearch* **3**(4): 303–312.

Walshe, K., Freeman, T., Latham, L., Spurgeon, P. and Wallace, L. (2000) Scope to improve. *Health Service Journal* 26 October, 30–32.

Winningham, M.L., Nail, L.M., Burke, M.B. *et al.* (1994) Fatigue and the cancer experience: the state of knowledge. *Oncology Nursing Forum* **21**(1): 123–136.

3

HOW TO DO A LITERATURE SEARCH

Sandra Colville-Stewart

- Identifying resources
- Planning your literature search
- Conducting your search
- Keeping records

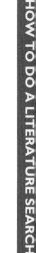

INTRODUCTION

As professional nurses our practice should be founded on research, and continuously evaluated and updated on the basis of research findings. The ability to search the specialist literature is an important skill not just for nurses directly involved in research, but for all of us. This chapter is not concerned with the process of literature 'review', defined as the intellectual evaluation or critique of the contents of published material (see Chapter 4), but rather with an effective strategy for finding the relevant literature, the literature search.

Examples will be drawn from the most important reference and indexing tools for nursing. If you need information from related subject fields, use the library and reference resource guides listed in the section on resource location. The basic literature search structure outlined here should be effective in any subject area.

STRUCTURE OF THE LITERATURE SEARCH

✔ Identify what information resources are available to you, pertinent to your topic.

Plan your literature search strategy:

Formulate a clear definition of your research topic.

Develop a list of relevant keywords/concepts.

Define the limits of your search.

 Do the literature search using resources such as library catalogues and indexes to journals, both computerized and printed.

✔ Organize your records. Decide which materials you wish to see, and locate copies.

Performing these steps in a systematic manner can save you time, frustration and probably money.

IDENTIFICATION OF INFORMATION RESOURCES

These resources include:

- Libraries and librarians
- Printed and on-line tools such as library resource guides, guides to current research projects, to theses, to the names of researchers
- Browsing of current nursing research journals
- Colleagues and professional organisations.

Keep these different resources in mind throughout your research project (Benton and Cormack, 2000).

Libraries

Libraries of use in nursing research include: academic libraries, including those of nursing and medical colleges, regional medical libraries, libraries of professional organisations such as the Royal College of Nursing, of charities and associations and some public libraries.

Two general guides to medical libraries in the United Kingdom are:

Directory of Medical and Health Care Libraries in the United Kingdom and Republic of Ireland 1997–8 (10th edn, 1997) published by the Library Association.

Guide to Libraries and Information Sources in Medicine and Health Care (P. Dale and P. Wilson (eds), 3rd edn, 2000; London: British Library).

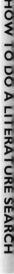

These directories are complementary: the second lists fewer libraries, but includes those of charities and similar organisations. New on-line services, such as that from RCN Wales at www.nursing-libraries.org.uk are also helpful.

To make the best use of any library, you need to possess some key information. For example, you should find out the following:

- Affiliation, location, telephone numbers, e-mail, Web address, opening hours
- Limits to access or borrowing privileges
- Subjects covered
- Types of material available
- Services available such as photocopying, computer searching, Inter-library Loan, and any charges
- Availability of service by telephone, letter, e-mail.

Much of this information is in library guides, and contacting the library in advance of your visit will save time. You might expect to need to visit or contact more than one library if your literature search is to be comprehensive. When you arrive at a library for the first time, spend a few minutes in orientation and in locating the librarians.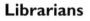

Librarians

These professionals are a fundamental resource in literature searching. The occasions when they can be of particular assistance include:

- When you are using a library for the first time and need information about its services and where tools are located; for example, ready reference materials, author/title and subject catalogues, classification guides, journal abstracts and indexes, the location of books, current and older journals, computer terminals and the databases available.
- When you are unsure of how to start looking for a topic.
- When you are searching for health statistics: a lot of data are available but often hard to locate.
- When you cannot find some specific item, or any material on a topic.
- When you want to be sure your search has been really comprehensive.

- When you want to do a computer search and need help in deciding on a database, selecting search terminology, or designing your search strategy.
- When you need material on Interlibrary Loan.

Library resource guides

There are several texts designed as guides to using nursing or medical libraries and to the bibliographic services available in them, including:

Resources for Nursing Research: An Annotated Bibliography (C.G.L. Clamp and S. Gough, 3rd edn, 1999; Thousand Oaks, CA: Sage Publications).

Guide to Library Resources for Nursing (K.P. Strauch (ed.) 1992; New York: Oryx).

Medical and Health Information Directory. Volume 2: Publications, Libraries, and Other Information Resources (L.M. Pearce (ed.), 11th edn, 2000; Detroit: Gale Group).

Information Sources in the Medical Sciences (L.T. Morton and S. Godbolt, 4th edn, 1992; London: Bowker-Saur).

These texts give information about all of the reference materials available. They include annotated lists of the appropriate indexing and abstracting services with dates, subject coverage, database information, etc. If your research topic expands beyond nursing into related fields such as health administration, psychology or education, these guides will supply the bibliographic information you need.

Guides to current research and researchers

If you are working for a higher degree, you need to be aware of the current research in your field, not only to avoid duplication, but also to enable you to participate in any network of researchers of similar interests. Several directories exist which can put you in touch, for example:

Current Research in Britain: Social Sciences, published annually by the British Library and covering medicine and nursing.

Index to Theses, with Abstracts: Accepted for Higher Degrees by the Universities of Great Britain & Ireland, published quarterly by Aslib.

Dissertation Abstracts International from the United States.

Royal College of Nursing's Steinberg Collection of Nursing Research as described by Smith (1983).

Specialist directories such as the annual *Midwifery Research Database MIRIAD* (1988–).

Browsing

Browsing the current textbooks and nursing research journals may also be useful. These include:

Advances in Nursing Science (1978–)

International Journal of Nursing Studies (1964–)

Journal of Advanced Nursing (1976–)

Nursing Research (1952–)

Western Journal of Nursing Research (1979–).

Miscellaneous

Colleagues, professional associations or charities, research institutions and conferences can be useful resources to help identify the most current research. You might also want to consult an Internet guide such as Nicoll (2000) for sites related to nursing research, grants, etc.

PLANNING YOUR LITERATURE SEARCH

Planning can be conveniently divided into three stages:

- ✔ Defining your topic
- ✔ Selecting relevant keywords
- ✔ Setting limits.

Define your search topic

The best way to do this is to write in one or two sentences, and as precisely as possible, exactly what it is you are interested in as if you were describing it to someone else. Asking yourself questions about the topic can help to clarify it. This exercise may seem too simple and obvious, but it is also too often omitted. Without a clear idea at the beginning of your literature search of exactly what you are looking for, you will be unsuccessful.

Sometimes this definition process will reveal that you are undecided or unclear on the exact nature of your topic. You may need to consult with colleagues or your supervisor, or do some preliminary reading in a textbook or research journal to help refine your ideas. Immediate success at this stage usually depends on how much you already know.

Once your search is under way, you may discover that your initial statement was too broad, too narrow, or even off the point. Successful literature searching requires flexibility at every stage and your statement can always be altered. Remember, though, that any such alteration may necessitate changes in your keywords or in the limits set on your search.

Develop a list of pertinent keywords/concepts

Having defined your research topic, you now need to break it down into components and identify any keywords, synonyms and related terms within each component. How many terms are used in each category will depend on your search needs.

Many sources, for example Roddham (1989), recommend that you draw up a diagram of these terms. Starting with each key element and its synonyms, branches are then drawn to lists of narrower terms, broader terms and related terms. An example, using the term 'diet', is shown in Figure 3.1.

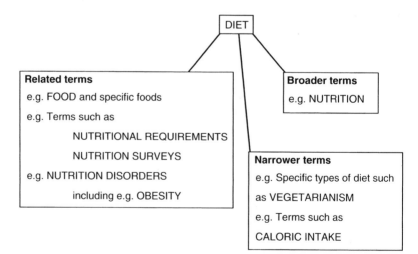

Fig. 3.1 *Draw up a diagram of terms*

This process is important for successful searching of databases and catalogues. As Treece and Treece (1986) point out, the tendency at the beginning of a literature search is to look only for studies exactly like the one you wish to do, which tends to be a frustrating and fruitless task. You can avoid such problems by thinking of related concepts from the beginning. Remember not to stray too far, however, or your search will collapse in a morass of irrelevant material.

Some ready reference tools can help in your search for keywords. There are several fine medical dictionaries and others with an emphasis on nursing such as:

Mosby's Medical, Nursing & Allied Health Dictionary (5th edn, 1998; St Louis: C.V. Mosby).

Baillière's Encyclopaedic Dictionary of Nursing and Health Care (1989; London: Baillière Tindall).

Miller-Keane Encyclopedia & Dictionary of Medicine, Nursing & Allied Health (6th edn, 1997; London: W.B. Saunders).

Standard textbooks are also useful in providing the accepted definitions of terms.

Finally, you need to become familiar with the subject heading lists used by the bibliographic indexes in nursing. The most comprehensive of these is *Medical Subject Headings (MeSH)*, the list of terms under which articles appear in *Index Medicus*, the largest medical index, available in print or through MEDLINE.

The nursing subject headings listed in the thesaurus of the *Cumulative Index to Nursing and Allied Health Literature (CINAHL)*, are based on *MeSH* but with some one thousand additional nursing-related terms.

A second nursing-specific list is the 'Nursing Thesaurus' included in the annual cumulated volumes of the *International Nursing Index (INI)*. Based on *MeSH*, this thesaurus gives useful *see also* and *see related* cross-references for topics of nursing interest where the *MeSH* term is less specific.

It is important to understand that these lists represent a controlled vocabulary. Panels of editors select the chosen terms. For example, in *Index Medicus*, *INI* or *CINAHL* you will not find articles under the heading DRUG ABUSE; the chosen entry is SUBSTANCE ABUSE. Sometimes different indexes use different terms, for example: NURSING CARE PLANS is a heading in *CINAHL*, but not in *Index Medicus* or *INI*, the latter have a *see* reference to NURSING PROCESS and PATIENT CARE PLANNING. It is helpful to identify the chosen terms for each index that you use. The indexes also help in preparing your keyword lists by means of permuted lists

(*CINAHL*) and subject classification structures (*MeSH*) (see Norris, 1992, for a useful summary).

If you are having difficulty finding terms in the indexes remember some further points:

 The spelling usage may be American.

 Indexes use nouns, not verbal phrases.

Indexes tend to invert compound terms if this brings related concepts together. For example, in *MeSH* the term DIET is followed by a list of related headings, such as: DIET, ATHEROGENIC and DIET, MACROBIOTIC.

Access to your topic may require use of a subject heading with a subheading. The latter include such concepts as Education, Manpower, Nursing and Rehabilitation.

 American indexes cannot necessarily be expected to have precise headings for concepts with strictly British usage.

Terms used may change, to reflect changes in medicine and nursing.

Always keep your lists of keywords under review as your search continues.

Define the limits of your search

Remember that you may not be able to establish all limits at the beginning nor to leave them unchanged as you progress. Some of the issues to be considered include:

- The time span of your search. Usually searches begin with the most current material and move backwards. How far back you search varies with the currency of the topic, its specificity, how much literature is found, the purpose of your search and your deadline. Most current nursing topics probably require a three- to five-year search.
- The language of acceptable materials. Indexes/databases such as *Index Medicus*/MEDLINE include foreign language articles. You need to know how to identify these and then how to obtain them if you need them.
- Geographic limits. Are you only interested in research done in the United Kingdom?
- Any age-group limitations, such as adolescence, the aged.

- Extension into related disciplines. This may be necessary, for example, to follow up on theoretical perspectives and methodologies.
- Type and quality of material in which you are interested. Choices include: primary sources, written by the individuals immediately involved, such as refereed research articles; secondary sources interpreting the work of others, such as most textbooks and many review journals. You may also need to decide if you are interested in such items as case reports, theses and dissertations, technical reports and government documents, conference proceedings, leaflets, news media reports and audio-visual materials or computer programs. Moorbath (1993) gives a useful outline of the content of most of these materials.
- How much time you want to spend on your literature search. Again, this will depend on your purpose. Estimates in the literature vary from 10% of the time allocated for a major research project (Lutley, 1994) to 25–30% (Mason, 1993). Remember that this time includes finding and reading all the materials.

THE LITERATURE SEARCH

Usually this involves consulting library catalogues and the indexing and/or abstracting services, as database or print, selected as the most appropriate for your subject and materials of interest.

Library catalogues

These may be in card, microfiche, microfilm or computer format. Remember that national catalogues such as that of the National Library of Medicine in Bethesda, Maryland, and other academic medical/nursing libraries are now available on-line.

The content of books may be older than that of recent journals, but is not necessarily out of date. Textbooks are often the best source for discussions of theory, hypotheses current in a field, conceptual frameworks and models. They may supply the names of key researchers, give citations to classic articles, and provide baseline bibliographies. Library catalogues also give information about materials such as conference proceedings, reports and audio-visuals which may not be included in your selected indexing tools.

When locating specific texts on the shelves, you may want to allow time to browse the adjoining titles. Serendipity can be important in successful research.

Indexes to journals

To locate pertinent journal articles you need to consult one or more of the relevant indexing tools whether in print or as a database. For nursing, the major indexes include:

Cumulative Index to Nursing and Allied Health Literature (CINAHL) (1956–)

International Nursing Index (INI) (1966–)

British Nursing Index (BNI) (1994–) (incorporates RCN database 1985–1996)

Index Medicus (1879–) may also be appropriate.

Earlier indexes, such as *A Bibliography of Nursing Literature* covering the period 1859–1980, the *Nursing Studies Index* for the period 1900–1959, *Nursing Research Abstracts* (1968–1994) and *Nursing Bibliography* (1981–1998) may also be suitable for certain topics. You may also wish to consider databases in related areas such as *PsycINFO* (1887–) and *ASSIA (Applied Social Science Index and Abstracts)* (1987–). Complete listings can be found in library resource guides.

Before you start your search, read any introductory information about the index; each has a section describing its contents and policies (Box 3.1).

Box 3.1 *Describing an index*

- How the index is constructed, author, subject, permuted indexes, etc.
- The criteria for selection by subject and types of materials. For example, CINAHL includes allied health, INI does not. Some include new books and reports, theses, etc.
- A list of the journals indexed by full title with a guide to the abbreviations used. *Index Medicus* currently covers more than 3800 titles, CINAHL more than 800, INI nearly 340, BNI more than 220.
- The languages covered: CINAHL and the BNI are English language only.
- Any subheadings used, and their definitions.
- The timeliness of the indexing, and how frequently any database is updated.
- Computerised database information: access, formats available, dates of files, etc.

Every index can be searched by author. For a subject approach in the printed volumes, you need to be familiar with the individual subject heading lists, the different controlled vocabularies as used by each index.

Even if you plan to use the computer database, a brief preliminary search in the printed index can indicate if you are looking in the right index and under the correct subject headings. Beginning with the most recent printed volumes and working back in time, you will rapidly develop a feel for the quality, quantity and type of material available on your topic. If the topic is simple, found directly under a relevant subject heading, and all you need are a few articles or even one good review article, then this may be the end of your search.

Double check by locating some of the apparently relevant articles to be sure they really are what you want, since titles are not always an exact guide to content. The articles themselves may give you key-word clues, the names of useful authors and bibliographies.

Be systematic. A chart indicating the years and subject headings searched for in each index can be very helpful, especially if your visits to the library can only be short and intermittent.

Fortunately, of the thousands of computerised databases now available, relatively few are required in nursing research. MEDLINE was one of the earliest and can be searched back to 1966, CINAHL to 1983, while BNI contains articles from 1984. The time span of the database may be important for some topics. When you log on, verify which years of the index are being searched for you, it may not be the full file.

The database may be available on-line or on CD-ROM (compact disk, read-only memory). The latter is now the preferred form of subscription for many libraries. Regular updates are sent out on new disks but the information on CD-ROM is still not as current as that available on-line. Some useful discussions/comparisons of the current database options can be found in Norris (1992), Brazier and Begley (1996) and Hek *et al.* (2000).

If you are unable to visit the library, or have little time, many librarians will perform searches for you, for a fee. If you are new to computers and/or literature searching, this is a good time to consult with a librarian, even if you wish to do the search yourself.

To search a database you need to construct a search statement or, more usually, a series of statements. This is an exercise in Boolean logic with three basic controlling connectors: *OR, AND* and *NOT.* For example, in the search topic: 'The nutritional status of substance

HOW TO DO A LITERATURE SEARCH

abusers', the basic search statements might be:

> *Statement 1:* NUTRITION *OR* DIET *OR* NUTRITION ASSESSMENT *OR* further related terms.

The connector *OR* is used to broaden the search so that the computer does not just look for the term NUTRITION but for other selected related terms as well.

> *Statement 2:* SUBSTANCE ABUSE *OR* STREET DRUGS *OR* further related terms.
> *Statement 3:* 1 *AND* 2.

The connector *AND* narrows the search: the computer is now looking for articles which include *both* groups of terms. This can be represented by Venn diagrams (Figure 3.2). The search will select articles represented by the shaded area only. Three or more elements can be combined in the same way, each *AND* connector narrowing the search further. Language restrictions, geographic or age elements, and article type can all be used as qualifiers in this way.

Avoid using the *NOT* connector, it is too easy inadvertently to omit important material. For more information about constructing search statements consult the database manual, the help screens or summaries in sources such as Lutley (1994) or Roddham (1989).

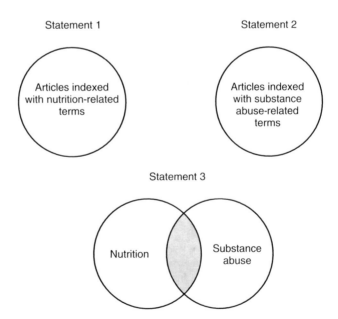

Fig. 3.2 *Searching a database*

Box 3.2 *Advantages and disadvantages of computer searching*

Advantages

- It allows great flexibility in designing your search strategy by combining and linking concepts. This is crucial when many keywords and complex combinations are involved.

- By allowing textword searching, the computer can bring precise and comprehensive results.

- The content is very current.

- By searching many years of the index database at once, a computer search can save you hours of time.

- Indexing terms and on-screen abstracts, giving clues to the content of articles, can save time in assessment of relevance.

- You may be able to download your references on to your own disk to store in your home computer.

- Access to journals and databases directly from home (MEDLINE, for example, is available free) increases the convenience further.

Disadvantages

- For some purposes, such as historical research, it is of limited use except as a source of secondary material via HISTLINE.

- Computer searches are not necessarily comprehensive.

- The search may not be 'instantaneous' if it is being done for you by a librarian or if your strategy is faulty.

- It may retrieve large numbers of irrelevant articles if not carefully planned and reviewed.

- It may be expensive.

- The differences between databases in terminology, search structures and software can be confusing.

- With limited numbers of terminals available in a library, you may have to wait to use the system or to make an appointment (Norris, 1992).

- Finally, as may be important at the beginning of your search, the 'serendipity factor' in computer searching is often lower than when scanning books or printed indexes.

It is often time-consuming to list all relevant terms in a related group and fortunately most databases have already pre-grouped related terms together listed on thesaurus screens. You can then search for all such terms using an *Explode*-type command.

It is also possible to search by free textwords or phrases as found in titles and abstracts, in addition to the subject headings of the controlled vocabularies. This is helpful when you are searching for very specialised or new topics. Word adjacency operators can also be used in textword searching to pick up desired terms occurring together, for example, where the words DRUG and ABUSE/ABUSERS are both present in a text. Truncation may also be helpful, for example using NURS* for NURSING, NURSES, etc., though it needs to be used with caution (Lutley, 1994).

Write your search statements out in advance before you sit down at the terminal. Adjustments may be necessary, of course, on the basis of your retrieval, but planning at the terminal can be time-consuming, expensive if you are on-line, and can easily lead to confusion if you have a long list of statements.

When your search statement is complete, scan a few of the articles retrieved, the terms used to index them, and any abstracts. You may then want to change or add some keywords, or alter your search statements. Your search will usually represent some compromise between precision and recall (Norris, 1992).

Databases can offer a choice of sorting format for your printout. Rather than in date order, the most recent first, you may want the list by journal title, for your convenience in the library stacks. You also need to decide what elements of the records you want printed. Indexing terms or even full abstracts, if available, may be helpful in selecting articles, but printing them can increase the cost of the search.

ORGANISING YOUR RECORDS

In organising your records, the most important principles are accuracy and consistency (Fox, 1982). Decide from the beginning which reference format you plan to use and apply it consistently. This will save time should you need to prepare a bibliography later. It will also help to ensure that you always record all the necessary elements of each reference. It is embarrassing and frustrating to be unable to find material a second time because you have made incomplete notes.

Whenever you locate any journal article or book, verify at the time that your original bibliographic reference was correct in all its details.

You may also want to gather more author information than is available in the printed indexes: full names, additional authors, addresses.

When you are recording your references, always use full journal titles. All indexes publish a key to their journal abbreviations.

Always note the sources of any reference: which database or index, the year and subject heading under which it was found. You will need this information should you need to obtain a copy through Interlibrary Loan. Also record the classification number under which you found a book, and the library (should you be using more than one) in which you found particular items.

In your literature review, or any work based on your literature search, never quote as if directly from a work you have not actually seen. If the quotation is from a secondary source, make that clear. The same is true of bibliographic citations.

If you want to take direct quotations from material, be sure to note the page numbers at the time. You do not want to have to find the source again.

Finally, you need to choose a format for organising your records. The traditional method uses index cards, which remains an excellent, flexible and portable system. Not only can you annotate them as you locate and read material, but the cards can be sorted into any convenient order, whether by author, by journal title, by date or by subject. Roddham (1989) and Pollock (1984) describe in detail how to set up such a file. Tait (1999) and Nicoll et al. (1996) describe and compare computerised reference managers such as Papyrus and Endnote which can sort, format and insert your citations into wordprocessed documents.

SELECTION OF MATERIALS

Always remember, as you scan the records retrieved, the criteria and limits established at the beginning of your search. Your immediate clues as to relevance will be: the title of the article and any abstract available; the journal itself, its type and quality; possibly the authors; and the subject headings under which it was found. The length of the article and its reference list may indicate depth.

The number of articles that you select is often dictated by the purpose of your search. Five highly pertinent citations may fill the need. A fully exhaustive search may require two or three hundred.

It is generally estimated that for any research topic 80% of references will be found in the major journals, but that the remaining 20% will be scattered (Roddham, 1989). Often, your need to find that elusive 20% dictates the complexity of your search.

HOW TO DO A LITERATURE SEARCH

LOCATION OF MATERIALS

As noted earlier, you may need to design some restrictions within your search statement so as to limit the number of articles you retrieve from hard-to-obtain or foreign language journals.

You will approach books, conference proceedings and other monographs via library catalogues; journal articles by the journal holding list of your library. Try to identify immediately those articles, books, etc., which you need to see but which will have to be obtained by Interlibrary Loan. Prioritise within this group, remembering that loans take time to arrange and may be expensive.

The Internet, e-mail and fax may speed up or replace Interlibrary Loan, but in some respects these developments have yet to reach full fruition. Although all major journals will eventually be available by full-text on-line or CD-ROM, as some are now, such advances may never include all periodicals and will probably never be retrospective.

Articles usually include an address for the author, who may be contacted directly for offprints or further information about research tools, etc.

CONCLUSION

Every time you approach the literature, whether to solve some immediate problem at work or to provide the anchor for a research project or funding proposal, your basic search strategy should be the same.

Always allow yourself enough time for all stages of the search, be well-prepared, well-organised, systematic and accurate. Good preparation at the beginning will save time later.

With experience, the planning stages speed up, database searching becomes more proficient, and a growing knowledge of the literature, and of library resources, accelerates selection and location. Major research projects will require frequent returns to the literature as new questions arise.

Remember that finding no articles on your topic can mean one of two things: either you have had a completely new and original idea, or you need to re-evaluate your search strategy (Treece and Treece, 1986).

KEY POINTS

✔ Identify the information available to you:

Research the libraries available to you.

Consult librarians.

Consult resource guides and colleagues.

 Plan your literature search:

Write a precise definition of your topic.

Take time to develop a comprehensive keyword list using subject heading guides.

Clearly define the limits of your search.

 Conduct the search:

If possible, familiarise yourself with the printed indexes before doing a computer search.

Plan your computer search.

Be aware of the advantages and disadvantages of computer searching.

Be systematic.

✔ Organise your records:

Be accurate and consistent in your record keeping.

Plan your record keeping in advance.

Select with care.

Allow enough time to locate and peruse materials.

COMMON PITFALLS AND HOW TO AVOID THEM

Pitfall	Solution
You arrive at the library only to find it closed After a long, hard afternoon's work, you realise the library has almost nothing on your topic	Check resource guides and/or telephone the library first for information on hours, collections, etc.
You spend two fruitless hours searching for some statistics: 'I know someone must produce these figures.'	Ask a librarian before you start looking.

HOW TO DO A LITERATURE SEARCH

You spend an hour doing battle with MEDLINE and finding little on what should be a simple topic, only to find it immediately in CINAHL	Take time to familiarise yourself with the scope of each database or index.
Your lovely long computer printout is ready: a mess of irrelevant articles	Define and plan your search carefully using keyword lists. Set your limits.
'It is such a great quote, but where did I find it?'	Keep accurate and consistent records. Note all pages for quotations at the time you copy them.
Your bibliography is due today but that key article has still not arrived by Interlibrary Loan	Allow enough time for seeing all your material. Check with the librarian how long an Interlibrary Loan may take.
Your thesis is nearly all typed when a colleague shows you a six-month-old article that refutes an entire chapter	Do a thorough literature search and keep it up to date.
You cannot find anything; the databases are too huge and daunting; the computer has turned into a monster	Do not panic. Ask a librarian for help.

REFERENCES

Benton, D.C. and Cormack, D.F.S. (2000) Searching the literature. In: Cormack, D.F.S. (ed.) *The Research Process in Nursing*, 4th edition. Oxford: Blackwell Science, pp. 89–102.

Brazier, H. and Begley, C.M. (1996) Selecting a database for literature searchers in nursing: MEDLINE or CINAHL? *Journal of Advanced Nursing* **24**: 868–875.

Fox, D.J. (1982) *Fundamentals of Research in Nursing*, 4th edition. Norwalk, CT: Appleton-Century-Crofts.

Hek, G., Langton, H. and Blunden, G. (2000) Systematically searching and reviewing literature. *Nurse Researcher* **7**(3): 40–57.

Lutley, S. (1994) Searching for information. In: Robertson, J. (ed.) *Handbook of Clinical Nursing Research*. London: Churchill Livingstone, pp. 15–29.

Mason, C. (1993) Doing a research literature review. *Nurse Researcher* **1**(1): 43–55.

Moorbath, P. (1993) The structure of the literature: varieties of journals and sources. *Nurse Researcher* **1**(1): 4–13.

Nicoll, L.H. (2000) *Nurses' Guide to the Internet*, 2nd edition. Philadelphia: Lippincott.

Nicoll, L.H., Ouellette, T.H., Bird, D.C., Harper, J. and Kelley, J. (1996) Bibliography database managers. A comparative review. *Computers in Nursing* **14**(1): 45–56.

Norris, C. (1992) Online and CD-ROM sources of information retrieval. In: Morton, L.T. and Godbolt, S. (eds) *Information Sources in the Medical Sciences*, 4th edition. London: Bowker-Saur, pp. 87–108.

Pollock, L. (1984) 6 Steps to a successful literature search. *Nursing Times* **80**(44): 40–44.

Roddham, M. (1989) *Searching the Literature. Research Awareness. Module 4*. London: Distance Learning Centre.

Smith, J.P. (1983) Steinberg Collection of Nursing Research (Editorial). *Journal of Advanced Nursing* **8**: 357.

Tait, M. (1999) Using computers in nursing research. *Nurse Researcher* **7**(1): 17–29.

Treece, E.W. and Treece, J.W. (1986) *Elements of Research in Nursing*, 4th edition. St Louis: C.V. Mosby.

4

REVIEWING THE LITERATURE

Linda Crofts

- What does a literature review look like?
- Stages of evaluating research

'Initially it seemed an overwhelming task, particularly choosing which library or libraries to search. However, as time went by particular references came up time and time again which made me feel that I had covered the ground fairly well. There was always a fear that there was a vital reference that I had missed or overlooked.'

Alison Hill

INTRODUCTION

The previous chapter has shown the complexities of carrying out a literature search and the importance of planning adequate time to explore library facilities thoroughly. By now you are stacking up a very neat pile of photocopied articles all ready to read and review. But how do you know if what you are reading is any good? It is generally theorised that the reason nurses do not base their practice on proven research findings, or indeed challenge other health professionals in their decision-making, is that they lack the confidence and skills to critique research (Akinsanya, 1994; Nolan and Behi, 1995). This problem is further compounded by many academic research modules starting out with critiquing a research report and building up to 'doing your research proposal' as though the latter were more difficult than the former. In fact the opposite is true; critiquing a piece of research is actually the most difficult skill of all quite simply because the reader has to have such a broad knowledge base of research to appreciate all the approaches a research project can take.

Critiquing literature is a skill that comes with practice and, ideally, opportunities to discuss research articles with peers. Many clinical practice settings are now promoting the concept of 'journal clubs' as a means of encouraging research mindedness among practising nurses (Aspery, 1993). These can take a number of forms but commonly focus around a selected article, distributed to the group members in advance, which is then discussed and critiqued at the journal club.

When critiquing a research report there is always a danger that you will instinctively identify all the things that fall short in the research rather than noting what is good about it. No researcher gets it completely right and many journals encourage a 'warts and all' approach to a research account so that readers can learn from others' mistakes. It takes confidence to present an article for publication in the first place (see Chapter 11) and if nurses are to be encouraged to publish their work then a constructive approach must be taken when critiquing an article.

You will be expected to take a critical approach when writing your literature review in your thesis. The fact that an author's work appeared to have a flawed sample group or to omit a dimension of care which seemed to you highly relevant does not mean that you should not include it in your literature review but that you should state its shortcomings in your write-up. Equally, where a study appears very strong and robust and set within a theoretical framework that is complementary to your study, then you may consider the work as a focal point for your discussion.

WHAT DOES A LITERATURE REVIEW LOOK LIKE?

The depth of the review will very much depend on the nature of your work. If you are writing your thesis then clearly you need to conduct an in-depth review although you must take account of the overall word limit. Some academic institutions actually give guidance on the percentage that the literature review should be and its weighting to the overall mark, e.g. 20%. It is very difficult to say how many references constitute an in-depth review; as stated in Chapter 3, you are probably best advised to look at some previous studies to get a feel for how thorough the literature review needs to be.

Word limits also have an effect on published studies. If a journal has a word limit of 1500 words then the author may decide to condense the review in order to allow more scope for describing the actual study; for example, Salmon (1993) focused on the philosophical discussions around pre-operative anxiety and therefore the literature review was adequate but condensed. This is in direct contrast to a published *review*, which attempts to give a broad, over-arching account of the main issues related to the topic; for example, Brearley (1990) devoted an entire book to a literature review on patient participation.

Literature reviews should read like a well-rehearsed dialogue. Keep your main question in focus at all times and then take each topic or dimension of the topic in turn and present the main arguments for and against. Literature reviews are often peppered with linking statements such as 'on the one hand ...' and 'while there may be some evidence to support X argument, Y offers a different viewpoint'. You are also attempting to be critical in your review and therefore need to highlight the shortcomings of both individual authors and the general approaches taken to the topic to date; for example, 'while Smith and Jones both suggest that patients could benefit from this intervention, both studies were hospital based and did not include patients in the community'. When you want to cross-refer or make links between a number of problems it can be useful to refer back to your Mind Map (described in Chapter 1).

The use of quotations is also worth a mention. Quotations can be invaluable for illustrating a point but they should be used sparingly. Long quotations can detract from the point you are trying to make and also use up your valuable word limit. However, a short quotation used appropriately can really invigorate your literature review. Wherever possible use primary rather than secondary sources.

As highlighted in Chapter 3, keep meticulous control of your references. It is not unusual in a Masters degree study to consult two hundred plus references and marks are usually deducted if they are inaccurate. Card index systems are probably the most reliable. Remember that if you are intending to compile your reference list at the end of your writing up, rather than as you go along, then you need to allow about a week for this.

'I got into a really good rhythm for my referencing. Every time I used a reference I would pull it out of the card index. I opened up a separate file in my computer for referencing and when I reached the end of each section of work I would add that day's index cards in alphabetical order to the referencing file. I divided the card index box into two so that references I had used were filed at the front and those I hadn't stayed at the back. At the end of my thesis I just printed out my reference list from the referencing file and those references at the back of the card index which I hadn't used became the bibliography. I was enormously proud of myself for being so organised!'

Linda Crofts

Classifying your literature review

The scope of the literature you find to review is not likely to be confined to primary research studies. Neither is it necessarily the case that primary research studies are the most significant literature you find, particularly if the studies are mostly small scale and not very well designed. Equally you may come across a report compiled by an expert group which is highly significant to your review. So how do you go about assessing the worth of the literature around your topic? One way is to classify your literature into the following categories.

1. Published research

The most common way of accessing primary research is in a journal which contains mainly original research papers, for example, *Journal of Advanced Nursing; NTResearch*. Such journals are considered high quality and the research credible because articles are reviewed by experts in the field before they are published. Many research studies are either the main points of a thesis or funded research studies carried out in academic departments.

2. Secondary research

As mentioned in Chapters 1 and 2, the publication of a systematic review, often in the same journals that publish primary research makes a significant contribution to your literature review and can also provide many excellent references to pursue further.

3. Professional practice

Many of the articles in professional journals such as *Professional Nurse* have an evidence base to their practice based articles and most articles are also sent for review to an expert referee. However, the usefulness of articles in such journals is highly variable; while very interesting, some may be little more than anecdotal and while making a useful contribution to your literature review, are unlikely to be the key texts you consult.

✔ Dissertations and theses

Occasionally you may find a reference on a database to someone's unpublished thesis. These can be extremely good sources of primary research because the research methodology and findings will be described in some detail. The difficulty you may have is accessing the thesis which may be lodged in a library many miles from where you live and that you will not know how good the work is considered by an expert referee.

✔ Reports

Reports are compiled for many different reasons; perhaps as a result of an inquiry, to publicise a new policy or be of special interest to a membership group. While very useful in discussing contemporary issues of the day, they are often written by an organisation with a vested interest in its message so are not always particularly objective.

✔ Conference proceedings

These are collections of papers that have been delivered at a particular conference. As assessment criteria for presenting at a conference are usually quite rigorous, they can be invaluable sources of primary research and current practice.

✔ Textbooks

Textbooks remain the primary theoretical source you need to consult in your literature review. However, given the time it takes to write the book and a further year for it to be published means it is unlikely to be your most contemporary resource.

✔ Professional opinion

Many journals give over considerable space to both expert and professional opinion on issues of the day as well as first hand accounts of experiences in practice. While there may be no research base at all for such opinions, they do give you a sense of what some of the contemporary arguments are around your topic and may also provide you with the names and contact details of groups or organisations who may be useful to you.

In summary, while you should aim to ensure a significant proportion of your literature review comes from reviewed research journals and is primary or secondary research, there is also a place for case studies, reports on professional practice and anecdotal accounts which often makes your review more rounded and alive. Providing your critique acknowledges the type of article you have reviewed there is no reason why you should not include everything relevant to your topic whatever its source.

EVALUATING RESEARCH

There are a number of texts that describe the process of critiquing the literature (Hawthorn, 1983; Parahoo, 1985; Burnard and Morrison, 1994; Cormack, 2000) but few encompass qualitative and quantitative approaches. Below is an eclectic model which can be a helpful aid when critiquing for the first time.

☑ *Title*

Research titles should be both concise and informative. The title should clearly indicate the content and, preferably, the research approach used. For example: A comparative study of; An ethnographic approach to; A double-blind cross-over. Therefore ask yourself 'Does the title provide a clear and unambiguous statement of the topic under investigation?'

☑ *Author*

Ask yourself if the author has the appropriate background to enable him/her to conduct the study successfully; for example, a psychology or mental health background. Qualifications can be a useful indicator.

The author's place of employment can, if known to be a centre of excellence, indicate that the quality of the published research is likely to be high (although not a guarantee.)

Multiple authors may indicate that there was a need for specialist input at various stages of the study or that a team of researchers was led by an experienced researcher who probably attracted the funding.

☑ *Abstract*

If one is present, does the abstract provide a clear summary of the research, i.e. outlining the research problem, the methodology and significant results and conclusions? This is crucial when you are initially 'surfing the literature' to help you decide whether you want to read the rest of the article or whether it is not actually relevant to your study.

☑ *Introduction*

As a rough guide you can expect to find that in the introduction:

- The problem is clearly identified and addressed.
- The rationale for choice of topic/methodology is described.
- The limitations are stated, for example a pilot study, specific population sample, only from a nurses perspective, etc.
- Depending on the approach, the research question and aims and objectives or the hypothesis/null hypothesis are stated. Ask yourself whether this is consistent with the topic under investigation.

The aim of the introduction is to give you some direction as to what is coming next.

✔ Literature review

This part of the research report will give some indication as to how informed the author is about others' contributions to the topic under consideration. Omission of any references that are central to the research topic (for example, by not referring to Jennifer Wilson-Barnett in a study about nurses and patient education) should be treated with suspicion; either the review is incomplete and/or the author does not know the topic.

A complete and detailed literature review should inform the conceptual framework (i.e. the theoretical origins) as well as previous articles on the topic. The literature review should also include up-to-date references, i.e. this year.

✔ Operational definitions

Closely linked to the literature review is the operational definition of terms. Keywords and concepts should be clearly defined and set in context for the purpose of the study. For example, what does the author mean by 'patient'? Is this an adult or a child, in hospital or at home?

An example of a good operational definition might read: 'For the purposes of this study the patient is defined as any male aged between 25 and 65 who has been admitted to the local hospital with an initial diagnosis of myocardial infarction.'

✔ Methodology/design/methods

There is a difference between research methodology and research methods that is often not made clear in research reports. The methodology is the approach taken, for example, action research; the research methods are the tools by which the data are collected, for example, pre- and post-intervention questionnaires, focus group interviews and reflective diaries, and the design is how the whole thing hangs together. Therefore in this section the research approach should be stated clearly with identifiable underpinning theory. The design should be justifiable and a logical description of what the researchers planned to do and how they actually did it. Without this description it would be very difficult to conduct a meaningful critique or for the study to be replicated.

✔ Subjects or participants

This should have been covered in the operational definitions. If not, then they should be clearly defined in the text before the description of the data collection phase.

✔ Sample selection

Ask yourself the following questions:

- Who or what forms the population for the study and are they appropriate?
- How was the sample selected? Was it self-selected, selected as most convenient or randomly allocated? Is it a representative sample? Does the author justify the sample selection?
- Does the author justify the sample size? Qualitative studies can use quite small sample sizes allowing for in-depth investigation, whereas experimental designs usually use larger sample sizes and researchers may have taken statistical advice on the size for the results to be statistically significant. Often a researcher is restricted by the time and number of participants available and should own up if this was the case.

✔ Data collection

If justification for the research methods is not given in the Methodology section then it should be covered here, with reasons for choice of methods stated. Then check the following:

- Are the advantages and disadvantages of each method discussed?
- Have the research instruments been piloted for validity and reliability?
- Does the researcher describe the data collection process?
- Are any copies of the research tools provided in the appendix? If not, can they be tracked through the references?

✔ Ethical considerations

There should be evidence that approval from the ethics committee has been gained (if appropriate). The author should indicate that consent has been gained from participants and that confidentiality has been maintained. This can be achieved by stating explicitly that all names and places have been changed.

✔ Results

The reader should ask whether the methods of data analysis used were appropriate for the research methods. Some raw data should also be provided as well as the findings. Results should be presented in a clear, concise, precise and logical manner so the reader can follow the analysis trail. They should also be sufficiently complete and detailed to answer all the research questions posed.

✔ *Discussion*

All results should be discussed in relation to the original research question/hypothesis. The discussion should be balanced, objective and draw upon previous research findings and/or the literature review to explain, compare and contrast other results obtained. Any limitations and weaknesses in the research study should be identified (e.g. poor response rate) and, if possible, suggestions made as to how they might be overcome in the future.

✔ *Conclusion*

Conclusions presented should be supported by both the results and the discussion. They should be limited to the original purpose of the study.

✔ *Recommendations*

Researchers will often make recommendations for further study. They may also suggest implications for practice. The reader should ascertain whether such interpretations are practical, accurate and appropriate.

✔ *References*

References should be complete and searchable. They should be arranged in alphabetical or numerical order in a reference list.

✔ *Appendices*

These should be clearly marked.

First attempts to critique a research report using this framework are clearly going to be lengthy affairs and at times you may feel you are missing the whole point of the research by breaking it down into such small units. However, in time you will get a feel for what is a good study and what is not and can simply refer to a framework when you require extra guidance. It should also be noted that while this framework will hold good for most research, studies using some qualitative methodologies such as grounded theory and phenomenology may not subscribe to this order of events.

CONCLUSIONS

No research is perfect and the fact that a research project has some shortcomings does not necessarily make it poor quality. Research in the real world does not always go smoothly and researchers are human who make mistakes. Well-designed research that did not go according to plan is not wasted if it can be replicated in another study. The art of critiquing is to recognise the difference between well-designed research that did not go well and poorly designed research with wildly inflated results.

KEY POINTS

 There is no substitute for systematically reviewing the literature on your chosen topic; therefore allow ample time for this process. However, do not panic if you cannot find one elusive reference.

 If you are too broad in your approach you will have far too much literature to review, if it is too narrow you risk missing essential pieces of work. Keep your original question in focus and use your word limit to guide you.

 Critiquing a research article is a very sophisticated skill acquired through experience. Journal clubs can be one way of getting together with colleagues to perfect skills in critiquing.

Remember that no research is perfect and you are looking for strengths as well as shortcomings.

REFERENCES

Aspery, C. (1993) How to set up a journal club. *British Journal of Midwifery* **1**(1): 17–20.

Akinsanya, J.A. (1994) Making research useful to the practising nurse. *Journal of Advanced Nursing* **19**: 174–179.

Brearley, S. (1990) *Patient Participation: The Literature*. RCN Research Series, Harrow: Scutari.

Burnard, P. and Morrison, P (1994) *Nursing Research in Action*, 2nd edition. Basingstoke: Macmillan Press.

Cormack, D. (2000) *The Research Process in Nursing*, 4th edition. Oxford: Blackwell Scientific.

Hawthorn, P. (1983) Principles of research – a checklist. *Nursing Times* Occasional Paper, August 31.

Nolan, M. and Behi, R. (1995) Research in nursing, developing a conceptual approach. *British Journal of Nursing* **4**(1): 47–50.

Parahoo, K. (1985) Research skills: critical reading of research. *Nursing Times* **84**(43): October 26.

Salmon, P. (1993) The reduction of anxiety in surgical patients: an important nursing task or the medicalization of preparatory worry? *International Journal of Nursing Studies* **30**(4): 323–330.

5

CHOOSING YOUR METHODS

Jill E. Robinson

- ■ Choosing the right method
- ■ Pros and cons of different approaches
- ■ Matching the method to the question

INTRODUCTION

It is not unusual, when talking to people about research methods, to be confronted by a wall of anxiety and a dramatic fall in self-confidence from people who habitually make life and death decisions within their working lives. There are a number of reasons for this. First, compared with research in other fields, clinical nursing research is still in its infancy (Hicks, 1996). This may be because, unlike many disciplines, we have not adequately established the boundaries to define what counts as research and what methods are most useful in collecting data about the practice of nursing and its impact on patients. Much of our current research uses methods borrowed from the behavioural and physical sciences which may not best suit the research requirements of a practice-oriented subject (Allcock, 1996). We are therefore confronted with an enormous array of ideological approaches and methodological techniques to choose from. In addition, in order to make an informed choice, we have to know as much as we can about the total array in order to reject some approaches and techniques in favour of others.

Secondly, although there is much in the literature to suggest that nurses have for a long time recognised the importance of research in nursing practice (UKCC, 1986), it has only been in recent years, since nurse education moved firmly into mainstream higher education that research has become firmly rooted in the curriculum. This has meant that for most experienced practising nurses, gaining research skills has been far from easy.

Thirdly, nursing is attempting to establish and maintain its academic credibility with other groups of health professionals. This means that much of the research that is published is deliberately written in a style that conforms to the rules of academia. This is not always the most accessible way of describing what methods were chosen and why.

WHERE WE ARE GOING?

In spite of these difficulties, method selection remains a vitally important element of the research process. Failure to choose an appropriate method to meet the demands of a particular field of study or research aim can render a study meaningless. Methodological decisions therefore lie at the very heart of the research process and have to be addressed early in the planning stage. Timetable, access and resource issues will necessarily vary according to the methods chosen.

This chapter aims to describe in clear, relatively jargon-free terms, the process of selecting methods to support a research idea and where that process sits in the overall context of a research programme. It will:

- help you make decisions about the best methods for exploring particular research questions;
- provide you with some skills to help you negotiate the maze of arguments and debates about the relative value and credibility of various approaches;
- bring the whole process of making methodological choices down to earth.

The range of debates that currently exist in relation to research methodology are well represented in nursing journals and at conferences. Many readers will have come across debates about what elements of nursing practice can be legitimately quantified or debates about whether or not methods that focus on small samples or a few cases can inform nursing practice in general. A recent paper, for example, attempts to redress what it calls 'the academic "romance" with the new found orientation towards exploratory descriptive research' (Poole and Jones, 1996, p. 108). These debates might focus on the ideological, philosophical aspects of particular approaches and, although they are important and interesting debates, they are not always useful in solving the practical problem of deciding the most efficient and effective way of gathering the kind of evidence needed to best answer our research questions.

CHOOSING YOUR METHODS

CHOOSING YOUR METHODS

WHAT ARE METHODS SUPPOSED TO DO?

This chapter will not merely take you through a list of methods with uses and abuses pointed out at strategic intervals. It will take you through a problem-oriented approach to method selection, emphasising the elements of the research process which should inform your choice.

First of all, it is important to understand some of the basic functions that all methods have to achieve. Methods are the tools of the trade of research. Their job is to:

 collect the best possible evidence to support or refute a particular argument;

 minimise the risk of bias in the collection of evidence;

 be practical and efficient;

conform to certain ethical positions in relation to the collection of evidence from human subjects (Burns and Grove, 1987, pp. 335–359).

THE NATURE OF EVIDENCE

 The collection of evidence is at the heart of all research and the credibility of any piece of research is established through the strength or weakness of the evidence upon which its findings are based. Poorly designed research and inappropriate choice of methods are often responsible for weaknesses in evidence. An example of this might be to choose rating scales to measure a concept which is very hard to define and which has different meanings for different individuals. One might, for example, ask patients to rate their experiences of pain. One person's concept of 'very painful' might be different from another person's experience. Each might rate the pain as the numerical value 5 but this would mean something different in each case. If statistical inferences were made on the basis of measuring an ill-defined concept of pain then the evidence would be weak and open to question.

In discussing the nature of evidence parallels may be drawn with a court of law. Evidence is presented to a jury to support either the case for the prosecution or the case for the defence. There is usually evidence which can be presented for both sides. The jury must then decide which evidence is strongest in order to arrive at a verdict. It will judge the strength of evidence in a number of ways. It might ask how the evidence was collected. Was the person providing the evidence under any duress? Was the evidence obtained from an independent source? Were the techniques used to gather evidence reliable? These questions are just as pertinent to research evidence as they are within a court of law. Our peers and colleagues who are likely to read the products of our research are those who will rightly make judgements about the strength of evidence we present and their starting point will often be the appropriateness of the methods we have used for the subject of our research.

Evidence can take many forms. It can consist of ticks on a checklist, numbers of occurrences or points on a scale. It can consist of written descriptions, tape-recorded conversations or videotaped behaviours.

SOURCES OF EVIDENCE

Sources of evidence are equally numerous. Evidence can be gathered from what people say about their experiences or feelings. It can be generated by observing what people do and how they interact. It can be gathered from observing the environment in which people exist and from examining documents which refer in some way to the problem being explored.

Choosing appropriate methods is inextricably linked to the kind of evidence needed to answer a particular research question and to the nature of the intended sources of that evidence. In turn, the kind of evidence required and where it might come from is determined by the original aim of the study. In this way, ultimately, the process of choosing research methods is uniquely bound up with the particular aims of research.

The following list of questions shows the sequence of decisions you might make in the process of choosing your methods:

 What does the research aim to achieve?

✔ What kind of evidence will be most useful in achieving that aim?

✔ From which sources might the evidence be collected?

✔ By what means should it be collected?

METHODOLOGICAL APPROACHES

Having answered the first three questions you will probably be in a position to make a decision about the broad approach you might take to your research. A methodological approach is often determined by a number of philosophical and ideological orientations as well as practical considerations of research design. Different approaches will make different assumptions about the nature of truth and reality. They will have a different view of the role of the researcher and place different emphasis on the need for objectivity, validity and reliability.

Broad methodological approaches can often be confused with actual methods of collecting data. What then is the relationship between an approach and a method for collecting data? An approach can refer to the particular methodological orientation of the research project and implies the particular philosophical and ideological stance taken by the researcher in relation to the subject and the process of research. Methods, on the other hand, can be understood as the techniques used to gather data. They can be grouped into those that generate predominantly qualitative evidence and those that generate predominantly quantitative evidence.

The next section not only describes a range of methods which you might draw on in planning your research, but also shows in what ways methods relate to broad methodological approaches and, in turn, how these decisions might be driven by the particular requirements of real problems.

THEORY TESTING OR THEORY BUILDING?

What then are the steps to be taken to decide on your approach and the particular methods you will use to collect data? Starting from the research problem you must first decide whether you are aiming to test a theory or hypothesis or whether you are going to build or develop a theory or model from an exploratory study. Each of these two positions will suggest a particular kind of evidence upon which to base your findings and each will send you in a different direction in your search for a methodological approach.

Figure 5.1 gives some indication of the way in which the research process might differ in content according to whether or not you are seeking to test theory or to build it. The examples of methods provided in this model are not exhaustive and can sometimes be used in a variety of ways.

Box 5.1 simplifies this somewhat to show how different starting points can help determine the direction of your choice.

CHOOSING YOUR METHODS

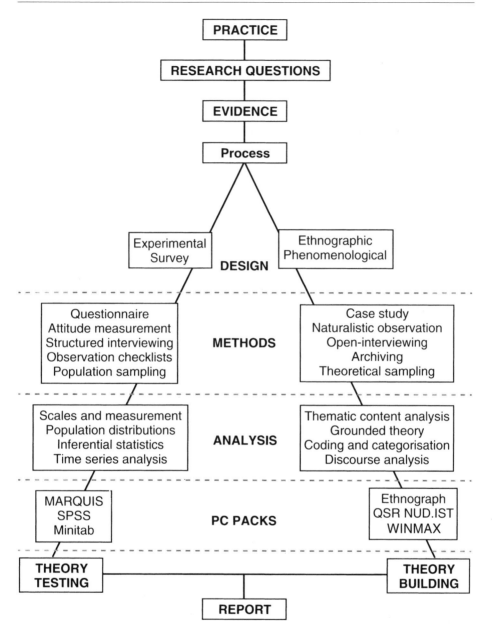

Fig. 5.1 *Theory testing or theory building*

Theory testing

You might have been reading a research report in the nursing press that suggests that patients are less likely to experience distress during uncomfortable examinations when they are given realistic information in advance about what they might experience. You are not

CHOOSING YOUR METHODS

Box 5.1 *Deciding on a methodological approach*		
Starting points	Theory/hypothesis	The field of study/data collection
Examples of evidence	Counts Measurements	Recorded speech Videotape behaviour
Examples of methods	Experiments Surveys	Interviews Naturalistic observation
Outcomes	Theory testing	Theory building

entirely convinced that the elderly patients you care for will feel reassured by knowing what discomfort they might experience and decide to see if this theory applies to your own client group. The starting point for your study is the theory expressed in the published research article. You might hypothesise that elderly patients undergoing uncomfortable examinations are less likely to experience distress if they are given information about what to expect.

 What kind of evidence might you need to collect in order to test this hypothesis?

You will obviously want to find some way of measuring levels of distress experienced by patients. You could, for example, ask patients to rate their feelings of distress on a numerical scale. Alternatively, you could observe the physiological signs of emotional arousal such as raised pulse and respiration rate. You might even observe elements of non-verbal communication that are associated with distress.

 Under what conditions will you collect evidence?

As soon as you have a clear idea of what your study will try to achieve, you must then plan your study to make it as controlled and unbiased as possible. You will probably want to compare the levels of distress experienced by two groups of patients. One group will have been given information (the experimental group) and the other will have been talked to about something unrelated to their care (the control group). You will try to ensure that all other conditions in both groups remain similar.

 From whom will you collect your evidence?

If you wish to test a theory you will want to test it on as many patients as possible in order to establish whether or not your results are clearly due to the experimental condition rather than to chance. You will want to seek evidence from patients who are undergoing the same examination. In this case you will be particularly interested in patients who are elderly. You might also want to make decisions about gender or mobility or other factors that might influence levels of distress other than whether or not patients receive information.

✔ How might you collect evidence?

This is where you choose your methods in the context of the information generated by the preceding questions. You might decide to record pulse and respiration rate for subjects immediately following their examination. You might decide to construct a standardised questionnaire to capture patients' perceptions of levels of distress. You might decide to administer the questionnaire face to face because the patients you are studying may be frail and find writing difficult.

✔ Some design issues for theory testing

Your research design sets out the way in which you intend to carry out your research. It includes your sampling strategy, your research tools and the procedures you will use to conduct your research. Your design must facilitate the control of bias, the selection of a sample which best represents the population you are trying to study and the rigorous measurement of the variables you are testing. The tools you use to collect data (e.g. questionnaires) must be as reliable as possible. In other words, the tools must be capable of producing the same results for the same subject in similar circumstances.

Theory building

Instead of testing a theory about a particular way of reducing the distress of patients when they are undergoing uncomfortable examinations you might want to explore how patients feel when they have such experiences and try to identify a range of ways in which patients might be helped. The starting point for your study in this case would be the real world of patients undergoing a particular examination. You know where you will look for information and from whom but you do not bring any particular hunches or theories to your study to invite any form of testing.

✔ *What kind of evidence might you need to collect in order to explore patients' experiences?*

You will want to collect information about the experiences of patients undergoing particular examinations. You will want to know how these experiences make them feel. This evidence might consist of descriptive verbal evidence of the things patients say they feel. It might consist of written notes of your observations of how patients behave during examinations. It might also consist of pieces of dialogue between the patient and staff.

✔ *Under what conditions will you collect evidence?*

In contrast to approaches which aim to test hypotheses, you will want to observe behaviour in natural conditions rather than standardise their experience in any way. You will be interested in any naturally occurring variation in the conditions under which examinations are carried out. You will encourage participants to talk freely and openly about their experiences. You will want them to feel there is plenty of time in relaxed circumstances so that they can express opinions and develop ideas.

✔ *From whom will you collect your evidence?*

Because this kind of data collection is time-consuming you will not usually be able to collect data from large numbers of patients. The emphasis in this kind of research is on the depth and richness of the evidence collected rather than coverage and generalisability. You will therefore probably choose a small group of elderly patients undergoing a particular examination. If you wish to gather verbal data you might decide to exclude from your study patients who are confused or who find speech difficult.

✔ *How might you collect evidence?*

Naturalistic observations are usually recorded in the form of field notes. The construction of field notes from naturalistic observation is an acquired and considerable skill. It requires the ability not only to record written information accurately, quickly and legibly, but also to notice a considerable array of detail and make sense of it on the hoof so that it can be written down.

In order to collect verbal data from patients you could use unstructured or semi-structured interviews. It is usual to tape-record responses wherever possible to capture the detail of what people are saying while staying alert to what is being said.

✔️ *Some design issues for theory building*

The design of an exploratory study which aims to build theory must take account of a number of issues. There is a need for control but this varies from hypothesis testing in that there is less need to control the environment and a greater need to control any preconceived ideas the researcher may have about what there is to be discovered. The emphasis here is not so much on objectivity but on open-mindedness. The study design must therefore facilitate disclosure and generate information about the particular rather than establish principles that generalise to the many.

TYPES OF APPROACH

The range of approaches can be divided into those approaches that tend to reduce the field of study into discrete variables which can be tested and measured and those approaches that tend to explore the field of study inductively with few preconceived notions about what will be discovered. The first group can broadly be described as quantitative approaches which tend to test theory and the second can be described as qualitative approaches which tend to build theory. The quantitative/qualitative nomenclature is derived from the kind of data generally produced by each approach. There are some approaches which span both of these orientations. An example of this is action research. This approach is generally participatory, where the subjects of research are actively involved in the research process rather than objectified and potentially devalued. It focuses on using research techniques to solve local, practical problems. Holter and Schwartz-Barcott (1993) propose at least three methodological orientations within the field of action research. These are:

- 'the technical collaborative approach' (predictive)
- 'the mutual collaborative approach' (descriptive)
- 'the enhancement approach' (both predictive and descriptive).

Through these orientations action research uses a range of different methods and can generate quantitative data, qualitative data or both. However, because of its tendency to focus on local issues it is rarely used to generalise its findings beyond the local context.

The following section gives some examples of particular methodological approaches which tend to be categorised as either quantitative or qualitative and uses examples of published research to illustrate some of the techniques associated with each.

Quantitative approaches

Quantitative approaches are largely based on the assumption that there is a single reality which can be uncovered or revealed by careful measurement. They assume that all human behaviour is open to measurement and that humans behave according to some universal principles which can be identified and used to predict future behaviour. The overall aim of quantitative research is to identify these general laws or principles of behaviour in order to predict and explain. The goal of the researcher in quantitative research is to be as detached from the subject as possible in order to increase objectivity and decrease the effect of personal values, feelings and perceptions. The key features of quantitative approaches are control, standardisation of instruments and numerical measurement. Types of quantitative research include survey research, quasi-experimental research and experimental research.

Survey research aims to describe variables within a given population by seeking evidence from a sample of that population. The relative strength of a survey often depends on the extent to which the chosen sample represents the population that is being studied. Standardised questionnaires are often used in surveys. Items are derived from the variables that are to be explored and responses to items usually take the form of scales or a choice of categories (Oppenheim, 1992).

The aim of experiments is to examine causal relationships. Most people associate experiments with laboratories where all variables other than the manipulated variable might be controlled. True experiments have three main characteristics:

- Some sort of manipulation or intervention
- An experimental group and a control group
- Randomised sampling.

Experiments that have these characteristics offer the most powerful evidence of all but are very difficult to design using human subjects and are rare in nursing research (Burns and Grove, 1987, p. 68). In nursing situations it is likely that there will be problems in controlling one or more of these characteristics. More common are quasi-experimental studies (Cook and Campbell, 1979), which examine causal relationships but do not offer the same level of control as true experiments. Most nursing studies examining causal relationships use some form of quasi-experimental design, as do most of the randomised controlled trials commonly used in evidence-based medicine.

Techniques for gathering quantitative data

Three of the most common ways of collecting quantitative data are to observe behaviour using a standardised checklist, to survey a sample of the population using a standardised questionnaire, or to measure performance following some experimental manipulation. Each of these techniques will be described in turn with reference to examples of published research.

Observation using a standardised checklist

You might wish to measure the frequency with which an element of behaviour occurs in a given situation. Routasalo (1996) examined the occurrence of spontaneous physical touching between nurses and elderly patients in a long-term care setting in Finland. An instrument was developed to record incidents of touching during specified periods of observation. Items on the instrument were generated by examining existing research on touching and by observing nurse–patient interaction in care settings. Each touch was recorded on simple pictures of the human body and contextual information written down. In this way the types of touch could be counted for each different circumstance recorded during periods of observation. The author highlights the importance of precise descriptions of what the researcher must observe in order to maintain reliability.

There are a number of important considerations in using this kind of observation. First, the behaviour to be observed and the conditions under which it is observed must be clearly and meticulously described to avoid unnecessary variation between observers. Secondly, the observed behaviours must be recorded in some standard way that can be represented numerically. Finally, the circumstances in which behaviour occurs must be clearly defined.

Survey using a questionnaire

If you wanted to gather data from a large number of subjects you might decide to construct a questionnaire. Although some questionnaires contain open questions which generate qualitative data, a questionnaire that can be coded numerically lends itself to statistical analysis and is a cost-effective way of achieving wide coverage.

Questionnaires were used in a study which showed that patients generally do not consider that they have adequate sleep while in hospital (Southwell and Wistow, 1995). Items on the questionnaire were generated from statements made by patients and nurses during unstructured interviews. Participants recorded their responses by marking a numerical scale, with each number representing a different level of experience. These scales are normally referred to as Likert scales. The researchers were able to seek the views of a large number of patients and nurses across three different sites. In all, 454 patients and 129 nurses completed questionnaires.

Measuring performance following intervention (quasi-experiments or pre-test post-test techniques)

If you want to carry out an experiment in which you measure the effect on behaviour of some intervention, you might try to isolate the effects of your intervention in one of two ways. You could either divide your sample into an experimental group and a control group, giving both groups similar experiences except that the experimental group will experience your intervention and the control group will not, or you could use a pre-test post-test design in which you measure some variable both before and after you carry out your intervention. This latter technique was used by McCain et al. (1996) to measure the effectiveness of a stress management training programme on 45 men who were HIV positive. One of the measures they used to compare the effectiveness of their programme was levels of $CD4^+$ T lymphocytes. Although the findings were not significant and the sample was small there appeared to be a trend towards a lower $CD4^+$ cell count in the control group, suggesting the possibility of a positive effect on immunological outcomes of the stress management programme.

The use of experimental methods requires considerable control of all variables other than the manipulated variable. This is a particular problem for research involving human subjects. Attempts to match control group subjects with subjects in the experimental group are fraught with difficulty given the uniqueness of human experience and the variation in the way individuals respond to particular health circumstances. Results from pre-test post-test designs can sometimes be challenged on the grounds that changes could in fact be due to maturation effects which occur simply because time has passed. McCain et al. (1996) used a control group to rule out maturation effects and to ensure that results were not merely due to individuals becoming more resigned to their illness and consequently less stressed.

Qualitative approaches

Qualitative approaches are largely based on the belief that reality varies for different people in different contexts. They tend to focus on the whole person as they interact with their natural environment rather than on splitting behaviour into researchable units out of context. The broad aim of these approaches is to discover reality as it is experienced by the subjects of research and to understand the meaning of experience from the subjects' perspective. The role of the researcher is to become involved in the field of study and use subjectivity and involvement to increase understanding. There are three main types of qualitative approach.

The *phenomenological* approach is often associated with the work of Edmund Husserl (Anderson, 1991). It takes as its starting point the total 'lived experience' of the subjects of research. The way in which individuals interpret their world and their subjective experience of it influence the way in which people interact with one another. This is the major focus in phenomenological research. One of its basic assumptions is that understanding human behaviour can only be achieved by taking an holistic view of people in their total historical and existential context.

The *ethnographic* approach is similar in that it, too, attempts to take account of the whole person in the context of their natural world and explores the field of study through the perceptions and meanings of the subjects of study. The origins of ethnography, however, can be found in anthropology and its conduct involves the researcher participating in the everyday lives of a particular group of people for an extended period of time (Hammersley and Atkinson, 1983). The aim of ethnography is to understand and explicate the meanings for participants of behaviours and rituals within a particular culture.

Grounded theory originated in the work of Glaser and Strauss (1967). It is often referred to as a method in research papers, but it could be argued that it is more a way of analysing data than a specific way of collecting it. It does, however, make some demands on methods used for data collection. Its substance offers a rigorous way of analysing data into categories and concepts. By exploring the relationship between concepts embedded in the data, theories about the meaning of data can be generated. It is most useful in making sense of data that are relatively unstructured and collected in naturalistic circumstances. One of its major premises is that data are collected as free as possible from predetermined theory, either in the form of assumptions held by the researcher or in the form of a conceptual framework to guide the research.

Techniques for collecting qualitative data

Naturalistic observation

Naturalistic observation is often closely associated with ethnographic approaches to research. It involves the researcher collecting evidence by observing subjects in their natural settings and recording observations as a set of field notes. Field notes might include evidence about the environment, the range of people present, the range of interactions observed over what period of time. They also record any unanticipated or unusual events as well as recording the mundane and ordinary events that occur.

Johnson and Webb (1995) used observation to gather evidence about how value judgements made by staff and patients can impact on decision-making. In this study, the researcher acted as a participant observer, working as a nurse on the ward while observing situations where nurses were faced with difficult moral choices. Observations were recorded as field notes and along with interview data were analysed using a grounded theory approach.

Unstructured interviewing

Unstructured interviewing is often used when the researcher does not wish to constrain the responses of the person being interviewed. This is often important when the field of research cannot easily be reduced to measurable variables and where complexity needs to be preserved in order to understand the problem.

Frederikson et al. (1996) used unstructured interviewing to explore family functioning and interpersonal relationships through the perceptions of women partners of Vietnam veterans in New Zealand. The reasons they give for choosing this method include lack of adequate theory and definitions in the field to produce valid instruments for large-scale survey techniques and the complexity of the social interactions involved in the impact of post-traumatic stress disorder on families. They refer to the need for 'greater density of information, vividness, and clarity of meaning' (Frederikson et al., 1996, p. 51) and chose a phenomenological approach to 'highlight the experience of veterans' partners within the context of their thoughts, feelings, and actions'. Interviews were conducted around an agenda consisting of a list of prime areas of interest. Each woman talked freely around the topics with limited intervention by the interviewer. Sessions were tape-recorded and transcribed.

Group-oriented techniques

There are a number of methods that use groups as a source of evidence and tend to generate qualitative data. Focus groups, for example, are discussion-based interviews which are facilitated by a researcher around a specific focus or theme. Often the researcher will use a topic guide to prompt the group and target issues of interest.

Group-oriented methods are increasingly being used to conduct participatory research (Heron, 1996). Broadly speaking, researcher and researched work together in equal partnership to pursue a particular research goal. The group might consist of a researcher and participants or all members of the group may act as both researcher and source of data. Rutman (1996) explored the policy and practice implications of caregivers' experiences of powerfulness and powerlessness. She used group workshops to generate data. Brainstorming techniques were used to explore the 'ideal' caregiving situation and critical incident exercises were used to generate examples of experiences of powerfulness and powerlessness.

There is no doubt that the use of group interaction as a source of evidence yields rich data. Concerns are expressed, however, about the lack of rigour with which these methods are used and the potential for these approaches to degenerate into nothing more than 'a well targeted and designed meeting' rather than a serious research tool (Breakwell *et al.*, 1995, p. 275).

CONCLUDING COMMENTS

This chapter has not given exhaustive details of methods and methodological approaches. There are many excellent texts which provide a thorough account of how to use particular methods and some of the most commonly used are included in the reference list. What this chapter has tried to do is demonstrate the process of deciding what methods you might use to explore clinical nursing research problems with reference to examples of published research. It should now be clear that each step in the research process is inextricably linked and that the collection of evidence is central to each step and is the critical element in making decisions about methods. As well as the range of textbooks that describe methodological techniques in some detail, there are other resources which researchers can draw on from time to time. The most important of these resources are the people around you who have particular expertise. Taking a team approach to your project is one way of marshalling other people's expertise and strengthening your project. It is also possible to contact the authors of published research papers if you wish to discuss their methods in more detail. Most researchers are only too happy to share their experiences with other researchers. Even the most experienced will turn to their peers for advice and ideas on a regular basis.

KEY POINTS

 Methodological decisions lie at the heart of the research process.

 The choice of methodology must be made early on in the planning process.

You must choose the best method to explore your research question.

You will need to consider:

- What kind of evidence to collect.
- Under what conditions will you collect evidence.
- From whom will you collect evidence.
- How will you collect the evidence.

 Utilise the experience of other researchers.

REFERENCES

Allcock, N. (1996) The use of different research methodologies to evaluate the effectiveness of programmes to improve the care of patients in postoperative pain. *Journal of Advanced Nursing* **23**(1): 32–38.

Anderson, J.M. (1991) The phenomenological perspective. In: Morse, J.M. (ed.) *Qualitative Nursing Research: A Contemporary Dialogue*. London: Sage.

Breakwell, G.M., Hammond, S. and Fife Schaw, C. (1995) *Research Methods in Psychology*. London: Sage.

Burns, N. and Grove, S.K. (1987) *The Practice of Nursing Research: Conduct, Critique and Utilization*. Philadelphia: W.B. Saunders.

Cook, T.D. and Campbell, D.T. (1979) *Quasi-experimentation: Design and Analysis Issues for Field Settings*. Chicago: Rand McNally.

Frederikson, L.G., Chamberlain, K. and Long, N. (1996) Unacknowledged casualties of the Vietnam war: experiences of partners of New Zealand veterans. *Qualitative Health Research* **6**(1): 49–70.

Glaser, B.G. and Strauss, A.F. (1967) *The Discovery of Grounded Theory: Strategies for Qualitative Research*. New York: Aldine.

Hammersley, M. and Atkinson, P. (1983) *Ethnography: Principles and Practice*. London: Routledge.

Heron, J. (1996) *Co-operative Inquiry: Research into the Human Condition*. London: Sage.

Hicks, C. (1996) A study of nurses' attitudes towards research: a factor analytic approach. *Journal of Advanced Nursing* **23**(2): 373–379.

Holter, I.M. and Schwartz–Barcott, D. (1993) Action research: what is it? How has it been used and how can it be used in nursing? *Journal of Advanced Nursing* **18**: 298–304.

Johnson, M. and Webb, C. (1995) Rediscovering unpopular patients: the concept of social judgement. *Journal of Advanced Nursing* **21**(3): 466–475.

McCain, N., Zeller, J., Cella, D., Urbanski, P. and Novak, R. (1996) The influence of stress management training in HIV disease. *Nursing Research* **45**(4): 246–253.

Oppenheim, A.N. (1992) *Questionnaire Design, Interviewing and Attitude Measurement.* London: Pinter Publishers.

Poole, K. and Jones, A. (1996) A re-examination of the experimental design for nursing research. *Journal of Advanced Nursing* **24**(1): 108–114.

Routasalo, P. (1996) Non necessary touching in the nursing care of elderly people. *Journal of Advanced Nursing* **23**(5): 904–911.

Rutman, D. (1996) Caregiving as women's work: women's experiences of powerfulness and powerlessness as caregivers. *Qualitative Health Research* **6**(1): 90–111.

Southwell, M.T. and Wistow, G. (1995) Sleep in hospitals at night: are patients needs being met? *Journal of Advanced Nursing* **21**(6): 1101–1109.

UKCC (1986) *A New Preparation for Practice.* London: UKCC.

6

WRITING A PROPOSAL

Maggie Tarling and Linda Crofts

- Writing a proposal for supervision
- Writing a proposal for funding
- Structure of a proposal:
  - for quantitative research
  - for qualitative research

INTRODUCTION

Once you have decided what you are going to research and how you are going to do it, you will then need to consider writing a research proposal. This is your opportunity to 'sell' your research idea to others. The purpose of writing a proposal can be as a means to obtain supervision for a Masters or PhD research project or to obtain a grant from a funding body. The objective is to state clearly what you aim to achieve and how you are going to do this. It is a useful exercise in any case, as it can help to clarify your thoughts about what you plan to do. The format and depth of the proposal will vary depending upon the reason for submission. If you are putting your ideas together in order to find a supervisor for your research project or PhD then the proposal may not be in any great depth, although saying this, some institutions will have different rules about the structure and content of the research proposal. However, if you are making an application for funding then your ideas should be well formulated and the proposal will need to be in much greater detail. What follows is a simple guide to completing a research proposal.

WRITING A PROPOSAL FOR SUPERVISION

The purpose of writing a proposal to obtain supervision is to give an indication about what you want to do and how you are going to do it. The most important thing to consider is whether you can realistically achieve your aims within the time and resource constraints you will be up against. Your supervisor will also need to assess that your research idea meets the requirements of the university course you are attending and that the research topic you have chosen 'fits' within the framework of the degree subject you are doing.

When you are at the stage of finding a supervisor you may find that your ideas are not clearly formulated. However, it is extremely important to identify a supervisor as early as possible. Expert supervision is critical when undertaking research for the first time and the relationship between supervisor and supervisee is outlined in Chapter 1. Therefore you may be putting a research proposal together before you have any clear indication about what it is exactly you want to do. It is critical to talk over your ideas with someone with research experience or the person you would like to supervise you as early as possible. Universities and academic departments will have guidelines about the submission of research proposals; therefore it is important to obtain these and more importantly to follow them. Moreover, the guidelines may also give some indication as to how the project will be 'weighted' (i.e. marking percentages) which you should note. If 40% of the marks are allocated for the literature review and only 20% for the data collection, then you will need to choose a topic and write a proposal which will optimise your chances of achieving the maximum marks.

Some universities actually count the research proposal as an assessed piece of work. In this case you need to have the proposal ready well in advance of when you plan to start your main research as you will naturally be waiting to see whether the assessor thinks your proposal is actually sound. Other universities place very little emphasis on the proposal and ask for a brief outline for the purposes of allocating a supervisor. You most probably will find that your ideas change over time as your research develops in the light of academic discourse with your supervisor and others. Many people find that the initial proposal bears little resemblance to the actual research project that is carried out. In many ways this is inevitable during the course of supervised research as there is also a learning process going on about the nature of the research process.

The basic structure of a proposal is very similar for academic supervision and grant applications. However, the grant application is in more depth and will also include information about costs. What follows is a guide for grant application proposals.

WRITING A PROPOSAL FOR FUNDING

Whereas a proposal for academic supervision may not be well formulated, an application for funding is very different. When applying to a funding body you will need to have prepared your ideas very clearly. Funding bodies are looking to fund research that is worthwhile and has a realistic chance of being completed in a reasonable time-frame; your research proposal is critical in communicating this. The funding body will want to see a clear definition of the research problem and its importance. Your choice of methodology should be clearly stated and should be the most appropriate one to be able to answer the research question or test the research hypothesis. You should be very clear about the research design and how you are going to conduct the research. There should be an indication that the research is in fact 'do-able'. To this end the funding body will want to know about the research backgrounds of those involved in the study. They will also want to know where the research will be conducted and what subjects will be involved, i.e. patients/clients, relatives, staff, and how you plan to get access to them. Most bodies will require ethical approval before you submit to them, so some of these issues would have been considered from an ethical perspective. Your proposal most probably will go out for critical review. It is therefore useful to consider the guidelines about reviewing the literature when you compose the proposal as these issues will be assessed by the reviewer (see Chapter 4).

Structure of a proposal for quantitative research

The following format is a guideline only. Many funding bodies will have their own application forms and guidelines. It is imperative when completing forms that you answer all the questions asked and if there is a word limit to certain aspects of the application, you must keep to them. If you do not comply with these simple steps your application will not be considered.

Abstract

The abstract is arguably the most important and the most difficult section to write. This will be the first section to be read and can influence whether the rest of the document is worth reading. Getting this right is therefore important. You will need to state the problem, why it is important and how you are going to tackle it. It will need to be very clear and brief. The difficulty arises because this section has such a restrictive word limit. It is advisable to get guidance from someone with experience of writing these applications.

Background and purpose

Here you should outline a short literature review to put your work in context. You should ensure that you include work that is up to date and well known in your area, if it is relevant to your research. Leaving out a critical piece from the review will communicate a lack of care on your part. You should also state the aims of your research very clearly. This is your opportunity to 'sell' your research, to indicate why your research is worth doing, why it is important and how relevant it is. It can also help your case if you can identify the potential impact that the results of your research will have on practice.

Design

Here you need to state how you are going to achieve your aims. You will need to state what type of subjects you will recruit, and what sort of methodology you will use. The methodology should be linked very clearly to your aims or hypothesis and should be the most appropriate to achieve your aims. You will also need to show which statistical tests you will use on the data and which framework you will use to analyse qualitative data. This issue needs careful consideration during the planning stage if you have chosen an experimental design. It is not good enough to have some vague notion about what you are going to do with the data once you have collected it.

Financial costs

Here you will need to give a breakdown of the costs of your research (see Chapter 7). You should include all the possible expenses you will incur in conducting the research. It is important to identify all the relevant costs as the funding body will only finance a research project that has a realistic chance of being completed. If you miss out a critical resource that you will need, you may jeopardise your chances of completing the study.

Structure of a proposal for qualitative research

There was a time not so very long ago when it was almost impossible to obtain comprehensive guidance either from universities or from funding bodies as to how to develop qualitative research proposals. An assumption was made that qualitative methodologies could simply manage a 'best fit' on grant application forms. Not only did this show a complete lack of understanding on the part of the host organisations about the nature of qualitative methods of inquiry but also clearly left qualitative proposals at a considerable disadvantage for funding because they did not neatly fit all the boxes on the form. There has also been some debate as to whether it is fair to have equal word limits for qualitative and quantitative work when, by its very descriptive nature, qualitative research is often lengthier. However, this state of affairs has improved considerably over the last few years and most funding bodies and universities offer guidance for qualitative as well as empirical studies. The NHS Centre for Reviews and Dissemination at the University of York has compiled guidance for reviews of qualitative work which can be accessed at ww.york.ac.uk. Below are a set of criteria developed by a team at the Royal Hospitals Trust which may be helpful in developing a qualitative proposal.

Criteria for the evaluation of qualitative research proposals

1 Are the methods of the research appropriate to the nature of the questions being asked?
   - Does the research seek to understand processes or structures or illuminate experiences or meanings?
   - Are the categories or groups being examined of a type which cannot be preselected or for which the possible outcomes cannot be specified in advance?
   - Could a quantitative approach address the issue better?
2 Is the connection to an existing body of knowledge or theory clear, i.e. is there adequate reference to the literature?
   - Does the work cohere with, or critically address, existing theory?

Methods

3 Are there clear accounts of the criteria to be used for the selection of subjects for study, and of the data collection and analysis?
4 Is the selection of cases or participants theoretically justified?
   - The unit of research may be people, or events, institutions, samples of natural behaviour, conversations, written material, etc.

In any case, while random sampling may not be appropriate, it is nevertheless clear what population the sample refers to.

- With particular reference to samples of time or ethnographic studies, how will they be chosen?
- Is consideration given to whether the units chosen might be unusual in some important way?

5 Will the sensitivity of the methods match the needs of the research questions?

- Does the method accept the implications of an approach that respects the perceptions of those being studied?
- To what extent are any definitions or agendas taken for granted, rather than being critically examined or left open?
- Are the limitations of any structured interview method considered?

6 Is the relationship between fieldworkers and subjects considered and is there any indication of how research will be presented and explained to its subjects?

- If more than one worker is to be involved, has comparability been considered?
- Is there any consideration of how the subjects might perceive the research?
- Is there a plan for conducting group processes if necessary?

7 Are planned methods of data collection and record keeping systematic?

- Will careful records be kept?
- Will the evidence be available for independent examinations?
- Will full records or transcripts of conversations be collectable if necessary?

Analysis

8 Is reference made to accepted procedures for analysis?

- Is it clear how the analysis is to be done?
- Has its reliability been considered, ideally by independent repetition?

9 How systematic is the analysis?

- What steps will be taken to guard against selectivity of data?
- In research with individuals, is it clear that there has not been selection of some cases and ignoring of less interesting ones? In group research, are all categories of opinion taken into account?
- It is sometimes inevitable that externally given or predetermined descriptive categories are used, but have they been examined for their real meaning or any possible ambiguities?

10 Will measures be taken to test the validity of the findings?
- For instance, will methods such as feeding them back to the respondents, triangulation, or procedures such as grounded theory be used?
- Are the data to be collected all relevant to the questions asked? (It should be noted that the phases of research – data collection, analysis, discussion – are not usually separated and papers do not necessarily follow the quantitative pattern of methods, results, discussion.)

11 Has the researcher's own position been clearly stated?
- Is the researcher's perspective described?
- Has the researcher examined his or her own role, possible bias and influence on the research?

12 Likely relevance and impact – are the results likely to be credible and important, either theoretically or practically?

Ethics

13 Have ethical issues been considered adequately?
- Is the issue of confidentiality (often particularly difficult in qualitative work) been dealt with adequately?
- Have the consequences of the research – including establishing relationships with the subjects, raising expectations, changing behaviour, etc. been considered?

CONCLUSION

Writing a proposal for funding is a very time-consuming exercise which is often undertaken within a short deadline. You invariably find out about available funds shortly before the deadline for application. As suggested in the next chapter it is often useful to have a series of research ideas in different stages of preparation. This can sometimes reduce the workload in making applications for funding. Given the amount of time and effort it takes to make a funding application it is important to follow all the instructions sent for completing the application. This includes sending the exact number of copies requested and filling out the form in the right colour ink or typeface. Missing out an essential piece of information may mean that your application is not considered and that all that hard work goes to waste. The application process is outlined in detail in the following chapter.

KEY POINTS

 Identify a supervisor as soon as possible.

 Carefully consider what you can realistically achieve within the time-frame available.

 Obtain any relevant guidelines and stick to them.

 When making an application for funding get help from some-one with experience.

✔ Make sure your ideas are clearly formulated.

✔ Ensure that you complete *all* questions on any application form.

✔ Keep within the word limits set by the funding body.

✔ Make sure you have applied for all the costs you will need to complete the study.

✔ Think about how you are going to disseminate your results.

WRITING A PROPOSAL

7

RESEARCH FUNDING

Joan Curzio

- Designing and planning for funding
- Current sources of funding
- Searching the Internet
- Importance of funding
- Obligations to the funding agency
- What happens if you do not receive a grant

INTRODUCTION

The issue of funding is the bane of many a researcher's life. Even when not having to find funds for their own salary, researchers are frequently forced to seek support for research supplies and assistance. This chapter hopes to give some help in identifying funding sources and some ideas about how best to approach them. In addition, a number of other issues related to funding will be covered.

There are innumerable sources of funding in the United Kingdom for research in general, but there are few sources specifically available to nurses or members of the professions allied to medicine (PAMs) for research that have a central nursing or PAM theme. The majority of such funds are limited, frequently ranging from a few hundred pounds to perhaps £10–30 000. However, this is changing for nursing and larger amounts of money are now being made available; for example, the Smith-Nephew post-doctoral research fellowship, announced in 2001, provides funding of up to £120 000 over three years.

Other money available for research has to be competed for with other professions including medicine. Nevertheless, some large–scale funding is available (even for nursing and PAMs). It is the strength of the application and the research 'track record' of the applicants, regardless of the profession of the applicants, that are of paramount importance when applying for funding.

DESIGNING AND PLANNING FOR FUNDING

Research support

It cannot be stressed too often or too strongly that it is essential to get help as soon as you start. Help can be obtained from numerous sources to assist in developing your grant proposal, although the availability of help will be influenced by where you work. Many universities have research officers or members of staff with a specific research remit who are very experienced in grant preparation and are charged with assisting fellow members of staff. Alternatively, you may know an individual in your university department who has successfully obtained grants and who may be willing to give you advice.

If you are not attached to an academic institution and are clinically based, you should contact your local research and development department or advisor or clinical effectiveness lead. Again, if you know someone in your clinical area who has carried out research, they may be willing to assist you. If an academic researcher is based in your clinical area, try approaching them for advice. Generally speaking, other researchers are usually willing to help where they can and, if not, are willing to tell you where you can go to get the help you need. Exploit the resources available to you in this way. You can save yourself a lot of grief.

If you want additional in-depth information before approaching local experts, there are a number of books that have been written on this topic; for example, Crombie and Du V Florey's *Pocket Guide to Grant Applications* (Crombie and Du V Florey, 1999). Many R&D and funding bodies websites have 'Helpful Hints' sections as well. A particularly well written and informative site is offered on the ReFund site at the University of Newcastle (http://www.refund.nc.ac.uk/RefundNew/Site/applications.htm). It even offers hints for when applying for European funding!

Project design

Before grappling with where to go for funding, you need to write a proposal (Chapter 6). Remember that your application must be able to withstand 'critical appraisal', so you should be familiar with the questions that are asked when critically appraising a piece of published research (see Box 7.1). These include ensuring that your aims and objectives are clearly stated, your methodologies reflect and allow you to be able to collect information from appropriate subjects

Box 7.1 *Critical appraisal questions (Fowkes and Fulton, 1991, with permission)*

- Is the study design appropriate to the objectives?
- Is the study sample representative of the population to be studied?
- Does the sampling method avoid selection bias?
- Does the sample size have sufficient power to answer the question?
- Are entry criteria and exclusions clearly stated and relevant?
- Are non-respondents dealt with appropriately, (i.e. their comparability to completion cohort)?
- Is the control group an adequate comparison group?
- Has matching and randomisation been carried out correctly?
- Are the measurements and outcomes being used valid and reproducible?
- If blinding has been used, has it been carried out as described?
- Does the study design address issues of compliance, dropouts, deaths or missing data?
- Does the study design address potential confounding factors?

to answer your aims and objectives. Also whether your statistical approach to the data you are collecting is appropriate and will generate results that will be able to answer your aims and objectives. Finally, many applications require you to say something about the potential benefits to the health services of your research proposal. These need to be clearly stated. If you wish to delve more deeply into critical appraisal Iain Crombie's pocket guide and Trish Greenhalgh's book on how to read a paper are very good (Crombie, 1996; Greenhalgh, 1997).

A clearly written, well-referenced and thoroughly thought out grant proposal will improve your chances for funding. Ambiguities and inconsistencies will be detrimental to your cause.

Project planning

Once your proposal is written, you will need to plan how best to carry it out. Many funding bodies will expect a project plan as part of any proposal they receive and it will also help you to clarify your project and identify any areas in which your expectations are overoptimistic. The project plan should outline the different phases of the project, what is entailed and how long you expect to take to complete each stage. There are various ways in which you can present this information clearly and succinctly. Two examples are given in Box 7.2 and Figure 7.1.

Box 7.2 *Tabulated layout for suggested broad project plan for a two-year project*

Months	Activities
1–3	Set up project Clarify and confirm data collection Obtain ethical consent if not already obtained Set up data input systems
4–21	Collect data Enter data as they are collected Begin analysing baseline data if appropriate
21–24	Complete data entry Complete data analysis Write up project report

---

	Project months*
	1 2 3 4 5 6 7 8 9 10 11 12 13 14 15 16 17 18 19 20 21 22 23 24
Set up project advisory group and set meetings	—
Clarify and confirm data collection	—
Obtain ethical consent if not already obtained	—
Set up data input systems	—
Train staff in data collection methodologies	—
Organise access for subject recruitment and data collection	—
Recruit subjects and randomise to group	———
Collect baseline data	———
Begin intervention	———
Collect follow-up data	———————————
Enter data as it is collected	———————————
Begin analysing baseline data if approriate	—————
Complete data entry	—
Verify statistical methods with statistician	—
Complete data analysis	—
Write up project report	-

*Once actual dates of project are known, the name of the months and year can be substituted

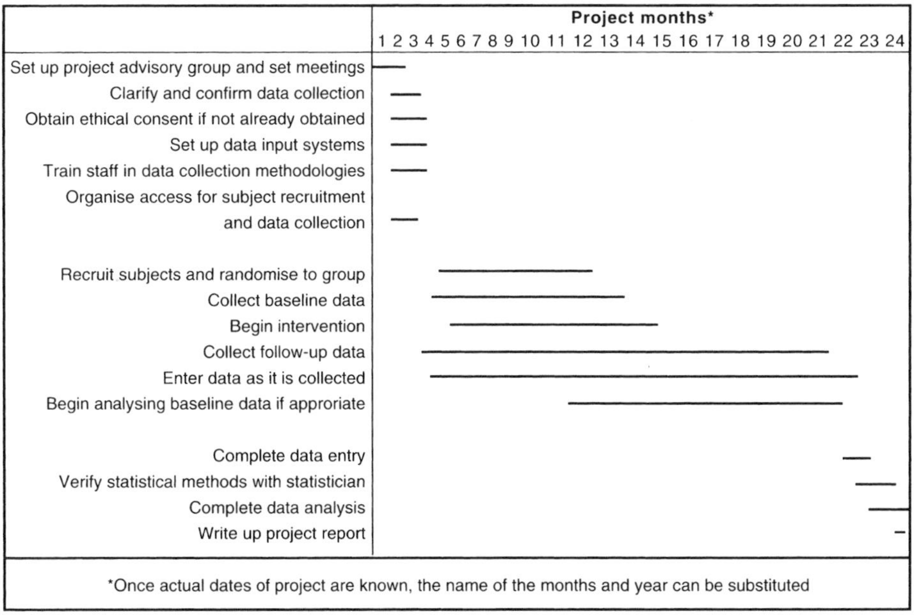

Fig. 7.1 *Gantt chart showing a suggested project plan for a two-year project*

It is essential to be realistic in your planning and to avoid over-ambitious schedules. For example, if you wish to conduct in-depth interviews with subjects and you estimate each will take one and a half hours, you will have to add in time in your plan for organising the appointments, travelling to and from, finding the address, writing up fieldnotes and transcribing the material onto your data analysis system. Therefore, it would be unrealistic to expect to be able to do more than one to two per day. In addition, you have to allocate time for interviews that are set up but do not happen. Thus if you want to do 50 such interviews, it will take at least 50–100 working days (10–20 weeks). If you only have 16 weeks in your plan for data collection, the problem quickly becomes apparent. You have to either extend the time in your plan, decrease the number of inter-views to be done or change your method of data collection. When planning your project, do your estimates, double them, and then you may have an approximation of the time it will actually take you to do it.

Project costing

Costing your project will tell you how much funding to seek. It is important to try to get this right. Again, continue to seek advice from an experienced researcher or researchers who agreed to help you develop your proposal. Otherwise you may find yourself out of resources before completing your study. Failing to complete a study can jeopardise your chances of further funding.

When costing your study you should identify all the activities and other resources that will be required to complete the work. Think through your entire project proposal and list what you will need to carry out each step identified in your project plan, revising your plan if you discover you require resources not previously noted. Then look to see what current resources are available to do some or all of the work. If you find you can support the entire project with local resources, you do not need to seek outside funding! A list of items commonly required when carrying out a research project and aspects of each needing additional moneys is given in Box 7.3.

Another costing issue if you are seeking funding from either a government source or a research council is identifying 'support costs'. These are the costs for any additional clinical care or treat-ment that would be undertaken within your study. These are funded from support funds administered by the research and development directorates in each region in England, the Chief Scientist Office in Scotland, the Wales Office of Research and Development for Health

Box 7.3 *Common research components to be included in costing*

Item	Components to remember to include
Staff salaries	'On costs', i.e. employer's National Insurance and pension contributions In addition, in qualifying universities, 45% indirect costs
Equipment	Any special equipment required for your study that is not available to you to do the work
Literature searches	Interlibrary Loans and photocopying
Paper and other stationery supplies	All research requires paper and lots of it
Travel expenses	Not only for researchers, but for subjects if they are asked to attend a centre for assessment
Office accommodation for researchers and other clerical staff	Including desks, filing cabinets, computers, Internet connection, and telephones Up to date computer hardware, software and printers Office supplies: printer toner cartridges, hardware maintenance Fax machine and telephone answering machine
Other related costs which may or may not be fundable depending on the grant giving body are:	Conference attendance Dissemination costs Higher degree fees
Management/advisory group	Travel and time to meet and discuss project
Depending on study design:	
Postal questionnaires	Not only paper, but stamps and envelopes for sending out and returning If large survey, consider getting help to stuff envelopes, apply stamps, open returns and enter data onto database
Laboratory work	Requires not only technician time and laboratory space but funds for assay kits, reagents, equipment and maintenance
Transcribing interviews	Can be greatly facilitated by clerical support (it has been estimated to take 8–10 hours of an audio-typist's time to transcribe verbatim one hour of taped interview)

and Social Care and the Department of Health, Social Services and Public Safety in Northern Ireland.

CURRENT SOURCES OF FUNDING

Traditionally, much of nursing and PAMs research has been conducted from academic centres and has not engendered a great deal of research support. However, health services research funding is available to all health care professionals. Therefore, nurses and PAMs are just as able to apply for such support as any other health care professional.

The shifts in the national political scene with devolution have subtly changed funding arrangements in the countries of the United Kingdom. Despite there being a 'Devolution Concordat on Health and Social Care' (http://www.doh.gov.uk/devolution.htm), which was agreed in 1999 and reviewed regularly, it is likely these changes will become greater over time. Keep in mind then that staff/organisations identified here as sources of information in each area may not be the ones best placed to tell you what is accessible at the time you are interested in obtaining funding. The current sources of funding at the time of going to press are described below.

Trust level funding

Many Trusts have small endowments that are available to staff for research purposes. The local research and development or clinical effectiveness staff and senior health service staff should have knowledge of these and their availability to local staff. Frequently, these funds are not advertised and it may take some effort to find out about them.

It is important to discover how the support fund (see Project costing section above) is administered locally and what, if any, help there is for new researchers. Again, it would be the local research and development officer/advisor/manager or clinical effectiveness lead that would know these arrangements.

Governmental funding sources

England

The Department of Health has a national NHS R&D programme which aims to identify NHS needs for research and commission research to meet those needs, generally through programmes of research that are managed by highly experienced researchers. NHS

Executive Regional Offices manage regional as well as national funding schemes such as the Health Technology Assessment programme. Project proposals are generally asked for under the government's targeted priority areas for research. The notices for deadlines for submissions are published on a regular basis in national newspapers such as the *Guardian* and the professional press such as the *Nursing Times* as well as appearing on their pages on the Department of Health website (http://www.doh.gov.uk/research/).

Currently, however, the Enterprise Award schemes hosted by each regional R&D department are the most accessible source of funding for the novice researcher. Both the primary and secondary care awards will pay up to £13 000 per year for up to three years which includes both course fees for research training and locum cover to release the practitioner from their day job to carry out their research. For those looking for funding to support PhD studies, the Health Service Research Fellowship is well worth exploring; an award of up to £110 000 for three years is available. Naturally, there are criteria that have to be met for both awards; contact your local R&D office for further details or look on the above website.

The arrangements for funding in England are currently being reshaped into two funding streams: NHS Priorities and Needs R&D Funding and the NHS Support for Science. The new researcher should be aware that the NHS Priorities and Needs R&D Funding is really designed to support experienced groups of researchers who have 'pre-qualified' before applying. However, as of the time of going to press, the NHS Support for Science stream is likely to have provision for research training, support and small project money.

Wales

The Wales Office of Research and Development for Health and Social Care (WORD), administers the research funds in Wales. They have established four university-based units across Wales to support health care staff wishing to undertake research. In addition they have a Health Responsive Grant Scheme and a Small Grant Scheme to which staff wishing to undertake research may apply. Further details can be obtained from their website: (http://www.dialspace.dial.pipex.com/town/road/xib80/calls.htm).

Scotland

The Chief Scientist Office, which is now part of the Scottish Executive Health Department, funds seven specialist research units based in academic departments across Scotland. It also offers responsive grants, and small 'mini grants' as well as having a Primary Care Research Fund. Larger grants have a two-stage process where a substantial outline is submitted for consideration and a full grant proposal done only if the first submission is acceptable. They offer postgraduate research studentships for which academics can apply to have a postgraduate student work with them on a specific project, as well as a research training fellowship for which health service staff can apply to obtain research training. The latest information can be found on their website at http://www.show.scot.nhs.uk/cso/

Northern Ireland

Since devolution, health in Northern Ireland has been the responsibility of the Department of Health, Social Services and Public Safety of the Northern Ireland Executive. Their R&D office is a directorate which offers similar support to that which is offered by the CSO in Scotland, WORD in Wales and the R&D directorates in the English regions. They offer studentships, a career development strand, and responsive grant funding including a programme for joint research project grants in biomedical sciences, health research and health services research with Ireland. http://www.rdo.csa.n-i.nhs.uk/rdo/index.shtml

Calls for proposals

At times, the government becomes more proactive in research by issuing a 'call for proposals' in an area relevant to its own health service research needs. These calls may entail only submitting a short two-page 'vignette', but others request full blown proposals with costs. One such call issued in 1994 for projects on the interface between primary and secondary care received 674 outline proposals, of which 103 were asked for full proposals and 54 of those were funded for a total of £6 million (Wisely and Haines, 1995).

Unfortunately, on many occasions, the time between first publication of the call and submission date has been relatively short at six to eight weeks. This can present quite a problem as research protocol development can take some time and effort. It is not always easy when you are working full time clinically or have other research projects under way. Therefore, it is a good idea to have projects in various stages of development. Then when a relevant call is issued, you may well have a project idea in a relatively advanced state of preparation, ready to be fully developed in the limited time-frame.

Finally, keep in mind that you do not need to be resident or working in a country to submit an application in another. Thus

Scottish researchers can apply to the Thames Regional Office when they put out a call on behalf of the Department of Health and English researchers can submit proposals to the Scottish Chief Scientist Office's calls.

The Medical Research Council (MRC) and other government-supported research funding agencies

The MRC offers funding for particular projects as well as personal funding for the development of research. Money is provided to the MRC by the government to generally fund basic scientific research. This can be a source for researchers, but the competition is very strong from all the professions, as well as from basic scientists, for these lucrative grants.

Other agencies that have governmental support for the research funds they distribute include the Economic and Social Research Council Learning Society Research Programme (ESRC), which funds projects in teaching and learning. A website that has links to UK research council websites is given in Box 7.4.

European moneys

The European Commission funds a biomedical research and development programme as well as another for the training and mobility of researchers. These require European collaboration (i.e. work to be carried out by researchers in more than one European country) and are not for the faint-hearted. However, it is a source of money and a sophisticated group could seek funding. Again, well-known names at an international level are more likely to succeed in accessing such funds. The EC website address is given in Box 7.4.

Funding specific to nurses

Funding specifically for nursing research and research education has increased in recent years. At one time in the United Kingdom there was only the Nightingale Foundation, Smith–Nephew Foundation, the UKCC, and the National Boards, with each offering grants of generally limited size. Now Smith–Nephew Foundation has increased their offerings, the Foundation of Nursing Studies funds work looking at getting research into practice and there is a new supporter of research receptive to nursing applications, PPP Healthcare Foundation.

The Nightingale Foundation continues to offer a number of scholarships that are administered for research education, and research

RESEARCH FUNDING

RESEARCH FUNDING

education travel bursaries and funding for specific research projects (http://www.florence-nightingale-foundation.org.uk/). The Smith-Nephew Foundation (http://www.snfoundation.org.uk/) offers research fellowships up to £5000 to support someone doing research towards a Masters degree, and up to £30000 to support someone already doing a PhD who wishes to be seconded for a year to concentrate on either data collection or analysis. In 2001, they established a postdoctoral nursing research fellowship of up to £120000 over three years.

PPP Healthcare Medical Trust was endowed in 1998 after the sale of the PPP Health Care group. At the time of writing, they estimated they had approximately £17 million to distribute annually. They have several themed programmes and offer a series of career development awards. Their website is at http://www.ppptrust.org/

The National Boards and the UKCC previously put out a series of calls for proposals for research that were published in the national nursing press. Like the Department of Health calls, these are in specific areas where the funding organisation has identified a need for information for their own purposes. Much of the research they look to fund is educational in nature. However, they have also supported studies that examine role issues. It is very likely that the new Nursing and Midwifery Council and related bodies will also be commissioning research. Unfortunately, these organisations tend to look to well-established researchers to carry out projects for them. If you are a novice and keen to try for one of these, seek out a well-known researcher for collaboration. They will, as previously stated, enhance your project and make it more likely that it will be considered seriously for funding.

The Royal College of Nursing (RCN) have an R&D advisor based in the RCN Research & Co-ordinating Centre, at the School of Nursing, Midwifery and Health Visiting at Manchester University who offers help and advice. They also have an extensive website which researchers find very useful (http://www.man.ac.uk/rcn/). The RCN Research Society (Scotland) offer a few small grants triennially to members.

Funding for PAMs

Funding for professions allied to medicine is even more limited than that which is available to nurses. Professional societies such as the Chartered Society of Physiotherapists offer occasional assistance. Professionals should contact their own professional society for the latest details of what is on offer.

Private trusts, foundations and charities

Other sources of funding are private trusts that have been set up by philanthropists and charities who fund research. Each will have an identified remit for the types of projects and the amount of money they are willing to give. These can be very specialised with many trusts only willing to support health workers in a defined geographic area or speciality. The charities, in particular, are interested only in projects relevant to them, e.g. cardiac rehabilitation project proposals are of interest to the British Heart Foundation but not to Cancer Care. Many sources of funding are listed in a variety of books that are published regularly, such as *The Grants Register* (Hackwood, 2001) and the *Handbook of the Association of Medical Research Charities* (AMRC, 2001). The Association of Medical Research Charities can be found online at http://www.amrc.org.uk/. There are also a number of other websites which list funding bodies (Box 7.4).

SEARCHING THE INTERNET

Those who have 'surfed the net' will know its benefits and limitations. However, if you have access or can get access, there are more and more websites being developed that would be of interest to researchers at any level. Keep in mind that material placed on the Internet has not been 'vetted' and the knowledgeable user considers the source, quality and accuracy of information obtained before using it. However, the site locations given here throughout the text are high quality, in the author's opinion.

Most 'search engines' (software programs that allow you to search the Internet) use the same principles as for searching bibliographic databases, i.e. you enter keywords or phrases of interest. Terms you might use are research funding, research support, nursing research, etc. A list of useful websites is given in Box 7.4.

THE IMPORTANCE OF FUNDING

Funding has more of a role in research than just paying the bills. Where you get your money provides you with further support and recognition for your work. Grants from prestigious grant-giving bodies look good on the curriculum vitae. Researchers are not only assessed on the number and quality of publications they have, but also on the number, type and size of research grants they have

Box 7.4 *A sample of Internet sites of interest to researchers*

Site name	World Wide Web (WWW) address	Description
REFUND	http://www.refund.ncl.ac.uk	Lists funding sources, requires subscription fee (but many universities and libraries subscribe)
Rdinfo	http://www.rdinfo.org.uk/	Lists 911 funding bodies offering 2283 different awards
NHS Executive Research Development	http://www.doh.gov.uk/research/swro	Southwest regional R&D directorate who provide information regarding R&D in NHS
The Research Page	http://ris.bournemouth.ac.uk/ sservice-depts/lis/LIS/Pub/res.html	General research site set up by a university
UK Research Councils	http://www.ja.net/janet-sites/ research.html	Lists the councils which fund research in the UK
Wellcome Foundation	http://wisdom.wellcome.ac.uk	Database of funding sources that can be searched in a variety of ways
European Commission	http://www.cordis.lu/	The commission's site

attracted. Frequently when you have already obtained a prestigious grant, regardless of where your name is on a list of holders for that grant, future grants are somewhat easier to obtain as you now have a 'track record'. Therefore, making yourself available to assist experienced colleagues with their research, collaborating with more experienced researchers from your own and other disciplines can be a pathway for developing your own expertise and 'fundability'. Wisely and Haines (1995) reported that groups with four or more disciplines represented had a greater percentage of their applications funded than ones with fewer.

OBLIGATIONS TO THE FUNDING AGENCY

Once a grant has been approved, the funding body will generally send the investigators their guidelines for completion of research. Each organisation has policies and procedures that are to be followed. If researchers divert too far from these guidelines, chances for further funding, or future funding of other projects, can be jeopardised.

Most funding organisations will require interim and final reports. In addition, if you find yourself 'getting into trouble' – that is, that you are going to be unable to recruit your full proposed complement of patients, or the preliminary data analysis has produced such skewed results that you will be unable to do your proposed data analysis, etc. – you must inform the funding body. They may well be able to help you with your difficulties; most research does not go entirely smoothly and funding bodies are aware that difficulties do arise.

WHAT HAPPENS IF YOU DO NOT RECEIVE A GRANT

Basically, life goes on. You have a number of options to consider once you have had a grant proposal rejected.

- Tear it up, throw it in the bin and never do research again.
- Look at it, consider any comments received from referees, seek further advice from experienced researchers, revise grant proposal and consider other funding sources.
- Carry out the research anyway using local resources shared amongst your co-investigators.

The last option may be totally impractical, as major projects require substantial input of staff time, which means funding.

If you are really perplexed as to why your proposal was turned down, most organisations are generally willing to discuss the matter more fully with you. However, you might be able to approach a trusted colleague for feedback so that the next time you tackle a grant proposal you will have a better idea of how best to approach it.

A FEW FINAL THOUGHTS

If you are just beginning as a researcher, start small and build up, working on yourself as a researcher as well as the work you wish to do. As previously mentioned, there are opportunities for small grants. Go after those and publish your results. Having results from pilot or smaller scale projects can lend a great deal of support to a larger project proposal.

Write papers and get them published, discussing issues in your area of interest. This helps verify your knowledge and position in your field. Finally, be willing to stick with your ideas, as research takes time.

RESEARCH FUNDING

CONCLUSION

In conclusion, the messages from this chapter are that obtaining funding is not easy but it is not impossible either and collaboration with more experienced researchers improves not only your chance of obtaining funding but your project overall. Therefore, you need to develop links with other researchers and begin to develop project ideas. Then when a call for proposals is issued for projects in your area of interest, you and your group will be in a far better position to compete for these moneys.

KEY POINTS

 Start small and build up your own expertise and research over time.

 Acquire as much information as possible about the funding source you are applying to, and their requirements. Make sure the group to whom you intend sending your proposal do actually take applications for the type of research you are proposing and that your request does not exceed their maximum amount.

 Multidisciplinary applications are far more favoured than individual ones.

It can be very helpful to have experienced co-investigators who will lend credibility, support and give high-quality input to your application.

 Your proposal needs to be as well thought out and presented as possible, with the aims, methods and statistical analysis all linked and the methods and analysis clearly identified to meet your stated aims.

 Keep abreast of the latest government strategies, policy statements and reviews.

Keep developing research ideas. If a call for proposals is issued you have a better chance of having an idea that can then be developed quickly into a more robust proposal than if you have to start from scratch with a tight time limit.

 Keep track of submission dates as they can come up far quicker than you think. Late applications are generally rejected without consideration.

REFERENCES

Crombie, I.K. (1996) *The Pocket Guide to Critical Appraisal: a Handbook for Health Care Professionals*. London: BMJ Publishing.

Crombie, I.K. and Du V Florey, C. (1999) *Pocket Guide to Grant Applications*. London: BMJ Publishing.

Fowkes, F.G.R. and Fulton, P.M. (1991) Critical appraisal of published research: introductory guidelines. *British Medical Journal* **302**: 1136–1140.

Greenhalgh, T. (1997) *How to Read a Paper: The Basics of Evidence Based Medicine*. London: BMJ Publishing.

Hackwood, S. (ed.) (2001) *The Grants Register 2002*. London: Palgrave (ISBN: 0333947290, cost £110).

AMRC (2001) *Handbook of the Association of Medical Research Charities*. London: AMRC. Tel: 0207-404-6454.

Wisley, J. and Haines, A. (1995) Commissioning a national programme of research and development on the interface between primary and secondary care. *British Medical Journal* **331**: 1080–1082.

8

ETHICAL ISSUES

Maggie Tarling

- Ethical principles
- Guidelines for ethical research
- Local Research Ethics Committees (LRECs)
- Multicentre Research Ethics Committees (MCREC)
- Ethical approval
- Applying for ethical approval

INTRODUCTION

With the introduction of clinical governance (NHS Executive, 1998) it is becoming increasingly important to ensure that practice is evidence based. As practitioners we must be able to justify the reasons for our practice. We must be able to review critically the evidence that is available about our practice. However, in the NHS this presents us with a problem. Patients' primary concern when coming into hospital is their own condition and its treatment. We have a duty to provide the best care for our patients, not only within the framework of our present state of knowledge but also to ensure that our knowledge remains the best in the future. We therefore have an obligation to the patients, the profession and society to develop nursing practice and knowledge and to keep this up to date. One very effective way of doing this is to be critical of our present practices and to strive towards a research-based practice. This is not easy and requires two fundamental things to happen: first, that nurses actually do research and secondly, that all nurses develop the critical skills to be able to evaluate health research in order to judge those findings for use in their own practice. So we have a professional and an ethical responsibility to ensure that our care of patients is the best now and in the future. But there is a tension in that statement. In order to develop we need to conduct research, but our patients come to us for care. They come into hospital expecting to be treated and cared for, not experimented on for the benefit of future generations.

So there is an ethical dilemma. We need to develop but equally we have a responsibility to the patients in our care.

These issues need careful consideration when planning research. Because of the complexity of research involving human subjects, Local Research Ethics Committees (LRECs) and Multicentre Research Ethics Committees (MREC) have been set up to evaluate the ethical dimensions of human research. Even if a study does get ethical approval and detailed information is given, one cannot obtain consent from a patient without a sympathetic and sensitive approach. Unfortunately, a book can only guide in this respect and cannot teach the subtleties of talking to patients about research. But we aim here to identify the important ethical issues that need to be considered when planning and conducting your research.

ETHICAL PRINCIPLES

It may be of some use to contemplate some basic ethical principles that have relevance to research; these are the notions of beneficence, non-maleficence and respect for autonomy. This is by no means a detailed review of these issues and further references are provided at the end of the chapter, but these principles are worth considering, as LRECs will use them in evaluating the ethical worth of your research protocol. Of course, there are other philosophies and concepts that individuals use in making ethical decisions. We now live in a multiracial society, so there are religious views other than Christian, which may have an influence on ethical decisions. These issues may have to be considered very carefully if any particular ethnic group is the subject of research. Research does not happen in a vacuum, and the researcher's own moral and ethical codes will influence the initial design of a project, but here we will focus on some basic principles that guide most LRECs.

Beneficence – to always do good

In general terms this means that one is morally obliged always to do good. Frankena (1963) described beneficence as the following:

1 One ought not to inflict evil or harm.
2 One ought to prevent evil or harm.
3 One ought to remove evil.
4 One ought to do or promise good.

ETHICAL ISSUES

The general interpretation of this principle in health care is that one must always do what is best for the patient and put the patient's needs first. In research terms this means that the needs of the patient come before the research protocol. Even if a patient has given informed consent to participate in a research project the paramount duty is always to consider their needs, even if this means breaking a research protocol and invalidating the results for that individual patient. No patient should have a treatment withdrawn when it is in their best interests to have that treatment. The needs of the researcher to conduct the study, and to get data in on a tight time-frame, must take second place to the needs of the patient. This moral injunction, to always do good, should sound very familiar to all nurses as this is the central theme of Clause 1 of the UKCC's Code of Professional Conduct.

Non-maleficence – to do no harm

The concept of non-maleficence states we should not harm another. This concept is extremely important when considering the ethics of conducting research with patients. Research should never do harm to an individual patient. There may always be a risk to any aspect of care or treatment; indeed some risks may be unknown. On balance the potential risks must never outweigh the potential benefits to an individual patient participating in a research study. If they do then the research cannot be conducted. This applies not only in situations where different treatments may be carried out, but also in cases where researchers have access to confidential information about patients. There should not be a risk that a patient's confidentiality is broken. The only situation where this might be acceptable is where it would be in the best interest of the patient or society or under court order to do so. This must be carefully considered because one must ask who is making the decision as to what is in the best interest of the patient. There may be an ethical debate as to whether the good of the many outweighs the good of the few. However, it is generally considered unethical to conduct research that may cause harm to an individual.

Beneficence and non-maleficence

To do good does not by the same token automatically guarantee that we may not do harm. Every treatment has a potential risk, both known and unknown. Therefore there may be potential benefits to a patient in participating in research but there may also be potential risks. LRECs generally evaluate the potential benefits versus the potential risks to the patients participating in research. The risks include not only physical ones from therapeutic treatments but also psychological problems from, for example, questionnaires. Questionnaires can be very invasive of an individual's privacy and may cause psychological upset or harm. There may also be risks of confidential information becoming accessible to inappropriate individuals. LRECs consider these questions very carefully. If the potential risks outweigh the harm to any patient then approval may not be given.

Autonomy

Autonomy is 'the capacity to think, decide, and act on the basis of such thought and decision freely and independently and without let or hindrance' (Gillon, 1986). If a patient's autonomy is to be respected, then health professionals must allow patients access to information in order that they can make rational decisions and have these decisions respected and acted upon. In the case of research, patients must have a choice as to whether to participate in a research project or not. It is generally accepted that it is inappropriate to include patients in research without their knowledge or consent. In order to consent, patients must have sufficient information to be able to make that decision. It is equally important that that decision is respected. One sometimes wonders why patients decide to participate in research. They come into hospital or go to their GP in order to get treatment. Many patients feel that they want to give some thing back. What we must always remember is that as health professionals we are in a very powerful position. Patients may feel that they have to participate in research because not to do so would jeopardise their treatment. It must be made clear to patients that they do not have to participate and that a decision not to consent will not affect their treatment.

Because of these problems ethics committees will insist on patients being given written information that they can understand and that makes the risks and benefits of the research very clear. It should also be made clear in writing that they do not have to participate and that their treatment will not be jeopardised if they do not consent.

In summary

The ethical issues of particular interest to LRECs are those involving the evaluation of the potential benefits and risks to patients. LRECs spend a lot of time ensuring that:

 patients are not being exposed to unnecessary or badly designed research;

 patients' rights to autonomy and confidentiality are upheld;

 patients receive adequate and understandable information on which to base their decision for informed consent;

 patients are not coerced into research.

GUIDELINES FOR ETHICAL RESEARCH

Why do we need guidelines?

Following the Nuremberg trials after World War II, the Nuremberg Declaration was published to try to avoid a repeat of the Nazi atrocities that had occurred. What was most shocking about the experiments conducted in the concentration camps was that both doctors and nurses had been involved – the very professions that were supposed to uphold the principles of the Hippocratic oath. This caused great public concern and questioning of these professions' ability to behave in an ethical manner and prompted the Nuremberg Declaration. Following this, in 1964, the 18th World Medical Association adopted the Declaration of Helsinki, which gave guidance to physicians conducting research on human subjects.

Even with the best will in the world, if you are a researcher you have a bias and an interest in conducting your research; you are not best placed to decide whether your research is ethical and will not cause harm to another. Therefore several guidelines have been produced to help researchers consider the ethical aspect of their research.

The Declaration of Helsinki

The Declaration of Helsinki is an important ethical document and sets out the guidance for physicians in biomedical research involving human subjects. The most recent amendment was introduced at the 41st World Medical Assembly in South Africa in October 1996. At the very heart of the Declaration is the principle that the health and safety of the patient is the prime consideration at all times.

The guidelines set out in the Declaration form the basis of ethical research and anybody involved in research must be aware of them.

It is also important that if practitioners are to be patient advocates then they too should be aware of these guiding principles. The Declaration forms the foundation for good clinical practice for research, LRECs and MRECs. The amendment adopted by the 41st World Medical Assembly in Hong Kong in 1989 states that: 'The design and performance of each experimental procedure involving human subjects should be clearly formulated in an experimental protocol which should be transmitted to a *specially appointed independent committee for consideration, comment and guidance*' (my italics). As a result of this amendment, most Health Districts and Trusts have an LREC that considers applications for ethical approval. It is interesting to note that although there is a statute that governs the conduct of animal research there is no such specific equivalent in law for research on human subjects.

GOOD CLINICAL PRACTICE FOR RESEARCH

The guidelines on good clinical practice for research set out in the Declaration of Helsinki primarily deal with clinical drug trials. However, these guidelines give a good framework for the conduct of good quality research in any area and the general principles are applicable to any research design. The principles of the Declaration of Helsinki and good clinical practice for research are used by LRECs and MRECs as the foundation of their review of applications.

Even though you may not directly be involved in a drug trial, it is useful to be aware of how new drugs and treatments are developed. As a practitioner you are in a more informed position and can act as a more powerful and efficient patient advocate if you are aware of good clinical practice for research and the processes involved with the development of new treatments. If you work in a teaching environment you are very likely to come across clinical trials. Clinical trials in humans have several phases in treatment development (see Box 8.1).

A phase I trial is generally conducted in a specialist centre and the aim is to investigate how the body absorbs and excretes the drug (pharmacokinetics) and the effect the drug has on the body (pharmacodynamics). Phase II trials aim to establish the safety profile of the drug and effective doses in a patient population. Phase III trials are usually large randomised controlled trials looking at how effective the drug of treatment is in a patient population. Phase IV trials are usually more interesting and often arise from clinical practice where clinicians will observe the effects of treatments that already have a

ETHICAL ISSUES

Box 8.1 *Phases of clinical trials*

Phase	Subjects	Aim
Phase I trial	Testing on healthy volunteers	Safety and pharmacological profile
Phase II trial	Testing on patients	Safety and dosing
Phase III trial	Randomised controlled trials	Safety and efficacy
Phase IV trial	Randomised controlled trials	Long-term safety and efficacy

licence, and feel that the treatment may be effective in a different condition or patient group.

Good clinical practice for research originally grew out of the pharmaceutical industry's increasing concern about research fraud. There were several cases where doctors had produced purely fictitious data. This is not to say that doctors in particular are prone to this sort of dishonesty but they have, within pharmaceutical research more of an opportunity to do so. The issue of falsifying data goes beyond the issue of dishonesty and in effect stealing, as these studies are paid for, but falsified results could mislead a company into thinking that their product is safe and effective when it may not be. Because of this, companies got together to produce guidelines on how clinical trials should be conducted and monitored. These guidelines cover the roles and responsibilities of all parties involved in a clinical trial. It is useful to be aware of this process. As time has gone on, each country had developed their own guidance. In order for a company to get a licence to sell a drug they had to comply with different guidelines from different countries. This was time consuming. Therefore an international committee we set up to harmonise this guidance. The ICH Harmonised Tripartite Guideline for Good Clinical Practice was adopted by the European Community in January 1997.

HUMAN RIGHTS ACT

Since the introduction of the Human Rights Act (1998) for the first time there is a potential for researchers to break the law. The Human Rights Act translates the 1950 European Convention of Human Rights into UK law for the first time. The Act comprises several rights or freedoms, expressed as articles, and are only applicable to

> **Box 8.2** *Potential implications of the Human Rights Act and research*
>
> **Article 2. Right to life** – *the right to life is protected in law and no one shall be deprived of life intentionally.*
>
> Everyone therefore has a right to access treatments that may be of benefit. The use of placebo groups will have to be carefully considered to ensure that patients do have equity of access to treatment. The implications of any research design that withdraws treatment from a patient group will have to be carefully explained.
>
> **Article 3. Prohibition of torture** – *includes deliberate inhuman treatment causing suffering and degrading treatment that puts an individual in a state of fear or anguish that debases the individual.*
>
> Researchers will have to ensure that they limit any potential harm that a patient experiences as a result of research. This not only includes physical harm but mental and psychological damage.
>
> **Article 8. Right to respect for private and family life** – *includes the right to confidentiality.*
>
> It is extremely important to consider the confidentiality of information about patients. Careful consideration will have to be made about accessing patient records for research. It has been known for researchers or companies to have access to information about patients who have been screened but not necessarily approached about a research study. There may be a case now that permission is sought before information taken at screening is given to a third party, be that a research department or a drug company.

public bodies such as the NHS. Box 8.2 shows several of these articles that may have relevance for research

The general principles in the Act are followed already in the ethical processes of good research. LREC and MRECs will continue to consider the dignity, rights, safety and well-being of research subjects. However, do not assume that because you have ethical approval your research is legal.

RESEARCH GOVERNANCE

The Research Governance Framework, currently in consultation and to be published shortly (Department of Health, 2001), will set standards for research conducted in the NHS. Research governance aims to improve research quality, promote good practice, reduce

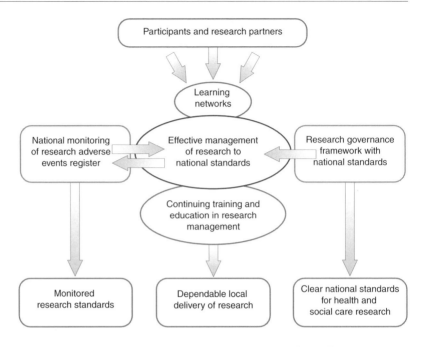

Fig. 8.1 *Research Governance Framework for Health and Social Care (Department of Health, 2001, with permission)*

adverse events, and prevent poor performance and misconduct. It is not only applicable to those who participate in research but also all levels of staff within the NHS no matter how junior or senior. Figure 8.1 sets out the Research Governance Framework for the NHS. It functions in a similar way to clinical governance (Department of Health, 1998).

I would suggest that you approach research governance in exactly the same way as you approach clinical governance: ensure the quality of your research by adhering to ethical principles and guidelines; ensure that you practice good science, no matter what research methodology you use; keep up to date with your subject and research methodologies; ensure that you have an obligation to prevent poor practice and performance; ensure that you are competent to conduct research.

PROFESSIONAL CONDUCT

Figure 8.2 identifies the main statements from the UKCC's Code of Professional Conduct and advisory documents that are relevant

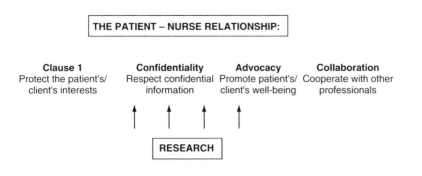

Fig. 8.2 *UKCC statements relevant to the conduct of research*

to research (UKCC, 1987, 1989, 1992). All of these statements are designed to protect the patient's or client's rights and buffer the patient from the worst violations of patients' rights that may potentially happen as a result of research. The most important statement is Clause I of the Code of Professional Conduct, which states that the nurse must always protect the interests of patients and clients. This must always come first. Confidentiality, account-ability and advocacy are also very relevant to research and these statements are quoted in Box 8.3. The UKCC include the specific criteria that ethical research should meet within their *Guidelines for Professional Practice* (UKCC, 1996) (see Box 8.4). All nurses should ensure that they have an understanding of research and the ethical problems associated with research, even if they are not con-ducting research, as they have a responsibility to protect patients' rights.

THE LOCAL RESEARCH ETHICS COMMITTEE

Research governance will set the standards for quality research in the NHS. Central to these standards is ethical research. All research con-ducted in the NHS needs to be referred for independent ethical review to safeguard the dignity and rights of individuals participating in research. There are also other important issues to consider as most funding bodies will not fund research that does not have ethical approval. Without ethical approval you may also find yourself in the uncomfortable position of not having indemnity insurance for your practice.

Box 8.3 *UKCC's statements with relevance for research (UKCC, 1992, with permission)*

The Code of Professional Conduct states that:

'Each registered nurse, midwife and health visitor shall act, at all times, in such a manner as to:

- **safeguard and promote the interests of individual patients and clients**
- serve the interests of society
- justify public trust and confidence
- uphold and enhance the good standing and reputation of the professions.'

The guidelines on confidentiality state:

'Each registered nurse, midwife and health visitor is accountable for his or her practice, and in the exercise of professional accountability shall:

- Respect confidential information obtained in the course of professional practice and refrain from disclosing such information without the consent of the patient/client, or a person entitled to act on his/her behalf, except where disclosure is required by law or by the order of a court or is necessary in the public interest.
- Where the person to whom that information is given is a nurse, midwife or health visitor the patient/client has a right to believe that this information, given in confidence in the expectation that it will be used only for the purposes for which it was given, will not be released to others without the consent of the patient/client.'

Exercising accountability:

Clause I of the code:

'Act always in such a way as to promote and safeguard the well-being and interests of patients and clients.'

Advocacy on behalf of patient and clients:

'Advocacy is concerned with promoting and safeguarding the well-being and interests of patients and clients.'

Collaboration:

'Collaboration and co-operation between health care professionals is also necessary in both research and planning related to the provision or improvement of services.'

ETHICAL ISSUES

Box 8.4 *Criteria for safe and ethical conduct of research (UKCC, 1996, p. 36, with permission)*

- The project must be approved by the LREC.
- Management approval must be gained where necessary.
- Arrangements for obtaining consent must be clearly understood by all those involved.
- Confidentiality must be maintained.
- Patients must not be exposed to unacceptable risks.
- Patients should be included in the development of proposed projects where appropriate.
- Accurate records must be kept.
- Research questions need to be well structured and aimed at producing clearly anticipated care or service outcomes and benefits.

You need to consider these criteria before submitting a research proposal to a LREC. You are expected to participate fully in the design process and this includes raising legitimate concerns when they arise. If no LREC exists in your area, it is important to refer to local policy for research.

Box 8.5 *Department of Health guidelines (1991, with permission)*

'The REC's task is to advise any NHS body on the ethics of proposed research projects which will involve human subjects. They are organised by district for convenience reasons, but it is the NHS body, be it DHA, NHS Trust, Family Health Service Authority (FHSA) or Special Health Authority (SHA) which decides whether the project should go ahead.'

'The REC must be consulted about any project involving NHS patients, fetal material and IVF monitoring involving NHS patients, the recently dead in NHS premises, access to recorded and use of NHS premises or facilities.'

The structure and remit of the LREC

The Department of Health issued guidelines in 1991 about the structure, the type of research and the general ethical questions that LRECs should address. Box 8.5 shows the Department of Health position on the type of research that the LREC should assess. The statement does make it clear that it is the NHS body where the

ETHICAL ISSUES

Box 8.6 *Recommended ethical questions LRECs should address (Department of Health, 1991, with permission)*

- Has the scientific merit been properly assessed?
- How will the health of the research subjects be affected?
- Are there possible hazards, and, if so, adequate facilities to deal with them?
- What degree of discomfort or distress is foreseen?
- Is the investigation adequately supervised, and is the supervisor responsible for the project adequately qualified and experienced?
- What monetary or other inducements are being offered to the NHS body, doctors, researchers, subjects or anyone else involved?
- Are there proper procedures for obtaining consent from the subjects or where necessary their parents or guardians?
- Has an appropriate information sheet for the subjects been prepared?
- Written consent should be required for all research (except where the most trivial of procedures is concerned); for therapeutic research consent should be recorded in the patients' medical records.

Box 8.7 *Research designs that require LREC approval*

- Clinical trials involving testing new drugs on patients
- Clinical trials involving new drugs on healthy volunteers
- Asking patients or relatives to fill in a questionnaire
- Interviewing patients or relatives
- Taking a blood sample from a patient
- Taking a blood sample from a healthy volunteer
- Asking hospital staff to fill in a questionnaire
- Interviewing staff
- Research on specimens and tissues/organs removed during an operation or procedure
- Research carried out for part of an academic course, e.g. degree
- Research involving patients' notes (without the patient being in hospital)
- Research carried out by another organisation on hospital premises
- Undertaking an observational study

research is being carried out that makes the decision whether the research goes ahead. This reflects the consultative role that the LRECs take in this process.

The Department of Health (1991) recommendations on the membership structure of the LRECs state that there should be 8–12 members on each committee and that it should include hospital medical staff, nursing staff, general practitioners and two or more lay persons. The lay view is particularly important in representing the public's interests. Box 8.6 shows the general questions that the LREC should consider with each application to them. These issues are very important to consider when designing your project and making your application to your LREC.

The Department of Health guidelines look fairly straightforward, but the reality is slightly different. Neuberger (1992) looked at the working practices and issues that LRECs had to face during their working life. She found that there is a great variability in the LREC's compliance with the Department of Health guidelines. Forty-three per cent of LRECs she looked at did not comply with the recommended numbers of members, either having less than or more than the recommended 8–12 members. There also seems to be a dominance of hospital doctors (52%) serving on these committees. Twelve per cent had no nurse representative and, most worrying of all, 34% had no or only one lay member. There was also a difference in working patterns. Committees met at varying times from monthly to twice a year. These are important points and have particular impact for nursing and multicentre research. With the predominance of hospital doctors serving on these committees, nurses have had problems getting approval, especially if their research is qualitative in design. LRECs spend most time considering quantitative drug trials as these are the most common application, and they are used to the issues raised by this sort of design. Multicentre trials also suffer because of the various practices that LRECs follow. It can be extremely frustrating when different LRECs have contrasting views about the same research project. To address this problem the Department of Health has now established Multicentre Research Ethics Committees (MRECs) in each region to assess protocols where the research will be conducted in five or more sites. However, you will still need to apply to each LREC once you have gained MREC approval (see Health Service Guidelines (97)23). Each LREC will expect an approval letter from the MREC when assessing your research. The MREC website gives useful information about multicentre research and an electronic application form (http://ds.dial.pipex.com/mrec/).

The issues the local research ethics committees consider

The LREC ensures that a patient's right to informed consent is upheld and that a patient's confidentiality is also respected, that they are not exposed to harm and are not coerced into participating in research. The LREC is the public's only guarantee that the patient's interests are protected when participating in research. It may seem obvious that ethical approval is required for testing new drugs and treatments on patients, so the list in Box 8.8 may seem surprising. It is equally important that patients' or staff's right to privacy is upheld; therefore issues about accessing patients' notes or information about staff must be considered by the LREC, especially where it is impossible to gain an individual's consent for this information to be accessed. The LREC should also consider the questions asked of patients or staff, either at an interview or on a questionnaire for purposes of research, as questions can be very invasive and personal, and though a patient or member of staff may choose not to answer questions they may be upsetting.

Box 8.7 lists different research methods that may be used in a health care context, all of which require approval from a LREC, though not all will require a full submission to the LREC. The more non-invasive studies may have other arrangements for approval, such as a letter from the chairman of the LREC.

LRECs generally do not review audit studies. However, there is a problem as it is sometimes difficult to decide when audit becomes research. Box 8.8 may be useful in helping you decide whether the project you are involved in is research or audit. Some LRECs will review audit studies if they involve the use of questionnaires. It is

Box 8.8 *The difference between audit and research (Clinical Resources and Audit Group, 1993)*	
Audit	**Research**
Aims to compare actual performance against agreed standards of practice	Aims to establish what is the best practice. Frequently explores new ground
Results apply only to the population examined	Results extended to the general population
Repeated to ensure changes are effective	One-off study

advisable always to consult the Chair of the LREC to establish whether or not you do need to make an application. This can save a lot of trouble later on.

Research design

It is the view of most LRECs that poorly designed studies result in sloppy research and therefore produce dubious or insignificant findings. You have therefore inconvenienced a large number of participants for no perceptible gain. This is just as true for qualitative as for quantitative research.

Qualitative research

There is a perception amongst nurses that it is difficult to get qualitative research approved by the LREC. The main criticism is that, as LRECs are made up primarily of medical staff, they reject qualitative research because they do not understand it. While this may have been the case in the past, the situation is improving as more nurses serve on committees. These nurses often have a good understanding of qualitative methods, as do an increasing number of general practitioners, social scientists and health service researchers who may all at one time or another serve on the LREC. The volume of applications using qualitative methods is increasing, not just because nurses are using qualitative approaches but because of the explosion of socially oriented health service research. As a result, LRECs should have a far greater awareness of qualitative research.

LRECs will reject a qualitative study if it is poorly thought out. It is not good enough to say that your study is phenomenology or grounded theory and therefore because you will be engaging in theoretical sampling you cannot provide the committee with any information about what you will be asking participants. What you can say is that when you have constructed your themes you will submit an outline schedule to the committee at a later date. Good qualitative studies are approved because the researcher has given plenty of background information about the nature of the problem and is clear about who will and will not be approached and what is expected from the participants. Issues of accessing the field, information for participants and consent are all sorted out and it is clear how the data are to be analysed. Even if it is a type of forwards and backwards (flip/flop) study involving both inductive and deductive thinking, this is all made clear in the purpose of the study. These studies get approval. It is well worth telephoning the administrator at the

LREC in advance to ask if someone on the committee who is familiar with your research methodology can give you some help with your application. It can save a lot of misunderstanding at the committee stage.

Coercion

Another important issue a LREC will consider is that of coercion. The LREC will consider whether staff, patients or students are made to feel, for example, that promotion, treatment or grades depend upon participation in research. Researchers are often in a powerful position in relation to their subjects. The researcher may not be aware of this, but it is an important issue. Patients are a vulnerable group. They are ill and have come in contact with health care providers expecting to be treated. It is extremely important that patients are not made to feel that their treatment would be adversely affected by not consenting to research. The process of consent and information given to patients is therefore of utmost importance. In fact, some LRECs insist that an independent witness is present when consent is asked of patients to ensure that the patients is not pressurised in any way. Though this is designed to ensure that no pressure is put upon patients there may be a problem with this. Often, it is a nurse who takes on the role of witness and he or she may feel pressurised into stating that there had been no coercion. Nurses should be very aware of the importance of this role and their obligations to the patient as an advocate.

Potential hazards

The LREC will consider whether or not any potential hazards that your research may expose individuals to outweigh the potential benefits. If it is clear that the hazards are unacceptable, then the research will not get approval. Treatments must never be withdrawn from a patient. If you are going to compare two or more treatments then the control group generally would be the normal treatment that the patient would expect to have. If it is obvious that the new treatment is much better than this it should not be kept from other patients. If it becomes obvious that the treatment is much better then the study should stop and the better treatment should be given. Equally, provision should be made in circumstances where it becomes apparent that the treatment is causing problems for a patient. The LREC will also consider the potential hazards to less invasive types of research. They will especially consider the importance of confidentiality.

Financial interests

Any financial interests must be made known as payment incentives may influence what research is conducted and the type of individuals agreeing to participate. Financial rewards may push individuals into participating in research when it may be in their best interests not to.

Confidentiality

The LREC will spend some time considering the issue of confidentiality. Researchers may have access to personal information about the patients or subjects taking part in research that may not be directly related to the research. Therefore researchers should always keep this information confidential and not disclose information unless it is pertinent to the study in question and only to individuals directly involved with the study. If information collected may be shown to other individuals this should be made clear to patients during consent. It is important that subjects' names and details are not stored with the data collected. Ideally, each subject should be issued with a number for identification. This information should then be stored in a secure place. Careful consideration should be made when storing audio- and videotapes of individuals. It is important that anyone involved in transcribing tapes is not aware of the identity of those talking. This may pose problems if videotapes are used. It is important to make a distinction between information that is anonymous and information that is confidential. For example, a questionnaire that includes personal information about an individual may not be anonymous, as the person could be identified. The information is then confidential.

Consent

LRECs have little power in policing the system. The central controlling factor in this process is that of patient consent. The consent process is therefore an extremely important one. Patients need to make a decision as to whether to participate or not with adequate information being made available so that they are fully informed and give their consent without pressure. The final decision is left to the patient. LRECs therefore spend some time considering the information that is given to patients so that patients have a good chance of understanding the risks involved in order to make the right decision for themselves. The researcher is not the best person to decide whether the research is ethical or not. There are too many issues, such as financial or professional ones, bound up between researchers and their research that their judgement may be clouded. It is therefore important that these issues are evaluated by an independent body.

If samples of either tissue or blood are to be taken, the situation must be assessed with care. Patients have a right to know what research is being conducted on any tissue or blood samples and consent is very important. These areas are often sensitive, especially when dealing with HIV, AIDS or genetic research.

SPECIAL CASES

There are some types of research where gaining ethical approval can be particularly difficult because of design, such as multicentre trials, or where the ethical issues are complex. You need to contemplate ethical issues very carefully when you plan to conduct research in vulnerable groups. These include children, pregnant women, those who are legally incompetent, such as people with learning disabilities or mental illness, or those who cannot give their own consent, such as intensive therapy unit (ITU) patients. There are strict ethical guidelines for these cases.

Multicentre trials

You may need to conduct a study over many sites. This is a particularly difficult and frustrating problem when trying to get ethical approval. All LRECs are independent, and separate applications need to be completed for each LREC area you intend to work in. Given that each LREC has different times of meeting, and different working patterns, and some insist on personal attendance, this can be a time-consuming process. One committee may pass your research but not another. This often happens as local conditions may be different and each LREC not only considers the general ethical issues but any local ones that may have a bearing on your research. If you are considering application to several LRECs it is important to plan for this very early on and allow time for getting approval. Following local guidelines becomes more important to limit any delays which may occur. If you intend to study more than five sites your protocol will have to be approved by the relevant regional Multicentre Research Ethics Committee (MREC) before being sent to each LREC for approval.

ETHICAL ISSUES

Children

It is considered unethical to conduct research on children where there is no direct benefit to the individual child. The Department of Health guidelines (1991) state that the consent of the parent or guardian for therapeutic research is essential.

> Those acting for the child can only legally give their consent provided that the intervention is for the benefit of the child. If they are responsible for allowing the child to be subjected to any risk (other than one so insignificant as to be negligible) which is not for the benefit of that child, it could be said that they were acting illegally. (Department of Health, 1991, 4.4)

LRECs will consider research on children very carefully before giving approval. Some ethics committees insist that the child should also consent to participate and where it is appropriate a written information sheet should be provided for children about the research.

Pregnant women

Given the problems with the use of thalidomide in pregnant women, research with this group is extremely sensitive. Research can only be conducted where there is a direct benefit to the mother and child and where it is impossible to conduct this research in any other group. There is some concern at the moment about the general exclusion of women of childbearing age from many forms of research. This has resulted in research results from a biased population and there is growing concern that we now have a growing body of evidence that may not relate to young women. This is a difficult ethical problem. On the one hand we cannot put potentially pregnant women at risk but equally we are faced with results from studies, especially pharmacological ones, which may not apply to this group. One has to balance the risks facing subjects and this is a difficult ethical question which will continue.

The legally incompetent

This group includes those who cannot give their own consent, such as the mentally ill and those with learning disabilities. The Department of Health (1991) guidelines state,

> research on mentally disordered people requires particular care and sensitivity bearing in mind that they are vulnerable and some

may not be able to give consent. There is a need to weigh the right of an individual to consent or refuse to take part in research, and the particular status of those unable to consent, against the need for research to advance the knowledge and treatment of mental disorder.

There are difficult questions as to whether consent by a relative would be sufficient.

The intensive care patient

Again this is a special group where individual patients may be unable to give their own consent. In this case assent is usually sought from relatives. This requires particular care as these patients are often very ill and approaching relatives for assent must be done sensitively at what is inevitably a very distressing time.

Prisoners

Prison inmates in hospital for treatment are particularly vulnerable when it comes to consent for participation in research. They are in a very powerless position and one cannot say that their consent would be given freely. They may feel pressurised by prison officers or may believe that participation would in some way count as good behaviour. It is therefore unethical to include this vulnerable group in any research.

APPLYING FOR ETHICAL APPROVAL

'I had only been in the post a couple of months when I had to produce a research proposal for the ethics committee. I knew it was going to be hard because someone had told me that they were having ongoing problems in having a study approved by them.

I thought a good start would be to seek advice. Not a good idea! The first person I asked was a consultant. His reply was, "ethics committee, ugh ... don't ask." The second person was a clinical nurse specialist whom I had heard was interested in

(Continued)

ETHICAL ISSUES

> research. "Yes", she said, "I did attempt a research project but when I saw the ethics form I decided to do an audit on the changes I had made instead." I decided I would just try and do my best.
>
> After a lot of stress and hard work, the proposal was ready for submitting. It was not approved. However, a month later it was accepted after a few explanations were given regarding certain points.
>
> *Allison Bell*

Planning

✔ Do you need approval?

If you are unsure about whether you need ethical approval in order to do your study you may contact the LREC and get advice. You may find that you do not need to submit a full application and that a brief summary of your proposal will suffice. However, you must check whether you need approval before you start.

✔ What is the LREC's deadline?

Find out how often the LREC meets. The frequency of LREC meetings can vary between monthly to twice a year. Most LRECs have a deadline before the actual meeting for applications to be sent in. It is important to establish what this deadline is. If you have a time limit to your research it is very important to establish the deadline as early as possible.

✔ Timing

Plan for at least two to four months for your research to be approved. It is likely that your research may get passed but only under certain conditions or after clarification if any aspect of your application is felt to be unclear. Therefore it is important when planning your research timetable that you allow extra time for queries to be answered before approval.

✔ Ethical issues

It is worth considering for yourself the ethical questions the committee will consider. Most importantly consider the potential risks to

ETHICAL ISSUES

patients and be very honest about this. Also consider what information you are going to give to your participants. If you are not going to give full information you must be able to justify this and indicate how you will debrief your subjects. It is not justifiable to deceive patients for the purpose of research and if you cannot give full information to patients at the time you must debrief patients after the study.

The Research Nurse's Guide to Ethics Committee Approval

Before any research can be carried out, ethics committee approval must be granted; it is therefore essential that research nurses not only know how to fill in a 20-page document but also understand obscure questions.

The following guidelines have been designed for beginners.

1 Always leave it to the last minute.

2 Always ensure a ready supply of coffee, matchsticks, pens and lots and lots of paper.

3 Always have a dictionary ready to decode the questions.

4 Always remember that you think better in the middle of the night, especially the night before the deadline.

5 Always remember that they need at least 35 copies of everything.

6 Always remember that you will have to clarify at least 20 points before final approval.

7 Always remember that no-one gets approval on the first submission, it's against policy.

8 Always remember that you are not in a hurry to start your research.

9 Always remember that the first six months of any research contract is spent getting ethics committee approval to start work.

10 Always remember that getting ethics committee approval is character building.

Finally, remember once you have ethics committee approval you will not have to do it again unless you change your protocol.

Amanda Armstrong

The application

✔ *The application form*

You need to obtain the LREC's application form. The form may vary between different committees, but it will generally address the issues covered already. The form may seem daunting at first as many are designed for clinical drug trials, which are the most common form of application. If yours is not this type of application most of the form will not be applicable. This makes the application easier, in fact, but you need to follow instructions carefully about the completion of the form. Not being careful at this stage will mean a delay later on.

✔ *What information?*

The golden rule about application to your LREC is to give more rather than less information about your research. Be very clear about what you plan to do. It is well worthwhile to include a protocol stating exactly what you are going to do. You should also include copies of any questionnaire you plan to use.

✔ *Plain English*

The style of language used in your application is very important. The best way of completing the application is to consider writing for the lay members of the committee. This means you need to explain all technical, medical and nursing terms in plain English. If your information is not clear then there will be a delay in approval. It may be useful for you to give your application to someone who is not medically qualified, a friend or family member, to see if they understand the application.

✔ *Patient information*

The use of language is even more important when designing the written information you will give to patients. Patients must understand this information very clearly. This might not be too easy if you have to explain terms such as placebos, randomisation, nursing models. Box 8.9 shows a list of common medical terms and suggested alternatives, from the East London & City Health Authority Ethics Committee guidelines. These may be useful when producing an information sheet.

It is important that certain issues are covered in the written information as a guide for the patient when considering whether or not

ETHICAL ISSUES

Box 8.9 *Common medical terms and suggested alternatives (East London & City Health Authority Committee guidelines reproduced with permission from the Ethics Committee)*

Terms to avoid	Terms to use
Placebo	Dummy tablet with no direct action on the body
Fasting	Having nothing to eat
Blind	You will not be aware of which treatment you are receiving
Double blind	Neither you nor your doctor will know which treatment you are receiving
Haematoma	Bruise
Pruritus	Itching
Catheter	Fine plastic tube
ml or g	Teaspoons, cupfuls, etc.
Randomisation	You have a 50:50 chance of …

Box 8.10 *Suggested questions a patient should ask when approached to participate in research (CERES, 1991, p. 4, with permission)*

- What will happen to me?
- Do I have to say yes?
- What will happen if I say no?
- Do I have to decide at once?
- What is the research for?
- How will the research help me?
- Can research be done on my child?
- What is a randomised trial?
- What is a blind trial?
- What is a placebo?
- Can I change my mind?

to give consent. Box 8.10 shows a list of questions from the Consumers of Ethics in Research leaflet, 'Medical Research and You'. They list a series of questions that the public should address when approached to participate in research. These issues are useful to consider when drafting the information sheet.

AFTER APPROVAL

If you do not get approval from the LREC you should be able to get information as to why your application was not successful. You might be able to take up the issues raised by the committee with the chairman. You might be able to meet the committee to discuss your research protocol and clarify any issues that have caused a difficulty. If you do not get approval it would be wrong to proceed without it. You may then have to reconsider what you want to do given the problems highlighted by the LREC.

If you have obtained ethical approval your responsibility does not stop there. Many LRECs require a written report on the progress of your research both halfway through and on completion. If there is any adverse event this should be reported to the LREC immediately and a decision should be made as to whether the risks to patients warrant the continuation of the research. If, as often happens once you are in the clinical area, you need to make changes to the protocol then you must go back to the LREC to get the proposed changes approved. The LREC may decide to have access to your research in order to assess that their guidelines are being adhered to. The LREC do not have policing powers, though they can withdraw ethical approval if they feel that patients are at risk.

'In the event, the project was approved with minor amendments only at one ethical committee, and approved unconditionally at the other. At the former committee the proposal was presented by a nurse who appears to be one of the few members of the 30 strong, medically dominated committee who understands and champions qualitative studies. At the latter committee, the proposal had the support of the consultant and was approved on the chairman's action.'

Anthony Pryce

OTHER ETHICAL ISSUES

There are many other ethical issues surrounding research that nurses may have to face. Nurses need to be more aware of the ethical issues connected with research and should consider their position very carefully. The UKCC's guidelines do help in defining the nurse's role in relationship with the patient. But there is a dilemma, in that the nurse has an ethical and professional imperative to protect the interests of patients but also has an obligation to cooperate with other professionals doing research. Clinical nurses are in a prime position to identify any problems patients may have when participating in a research project. It is important as a researcher to inform nursing staff about any research project before it commences as they have an intimate knowledge about patients and are in an ideal position to communicate between the researcher and the patient. The nursing staff should be aware of research being conducted so that the patient's care or a research protocol is not jeopardised. As a researcher it may be necessary to ask clinical staff to collect data. It must always be remembered that clinical staff's priority is to provide care and it is often better not to make these requests of busy clinical staff if at all possible. If you do, you must negotiate what is the best arrangement given the working practices of the area.

There are an increasing number of nurses employed by medical colleges as research assistants. It must always be remembered that these individuals are primarily nurses, not research assistants who happen to be nurses. Research nurses take their roles very seriously. The Code of Professional Conduct applies equally if not more so to these individuals. The interests of the patient always come first, and the research nurse is often the patient's best advocate in this circumstance as they have an intimate knowledge of the research process, the risks of any particular project and the potential impact that a research protocol may have for a patient.

In order to fulfil this role research nurses need a good working relationship with all levels of clinical staff they have contact with. They need to work closely with patients, their relatives, medical staff and other professionals the patient comes into contact with. But there may be conflicts of interest where research nurses are asked to do something which goes against their own ethical or professional values. This is a particularly difficult problem and is not easy to resolve and depends upon the level of communication that exists between the nurse and the medical team. An interesting ally might be a senior nurse, if you are lucky to have one in the district or Trust who has a responsibility for research. It may be of use to have contacts with any nurse who is a member of the LREC.

CONCLUSION

The present system is by no means perfect and there are many problems. Many people may not be aware of the need to get ethical approval for their research. If you consider the list of research designs that require approval (see Box 8.8) it is obvious that most research involving human subjects needs ethical approval to protect the public from the horrors that have occurred in the past. The LRECs are the public's only guarantee of protection. As a researcher it is useful to contemplate whether you would consent to participate in your own research, but these judgements, as we have seen, are not without bias. Therefore an evaluation by an independent body is very important.

KEY POINTS

 Remember that you are not the best person to evaluate the ethical value of your own research.

 Find out at an early stage how often the LREC meet.

Plan at least two to four months for approval; longer for multi-centre trials.

Follow the instructions for completing the application form very carefully.

Write the application form and the patient information sheet in plain English.

 Give more rather than less information about what you plan to do.

 Include all the questionnaires/interview schedules you want to use.

Include a detailed protocol.

Detail how you are going to get access to patients/subjects.

Consider how you are going to protect subject confidentiality and consider where you will store raw data.

COMMON PITFALLS AND HOW TO AVOID THEM

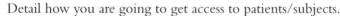

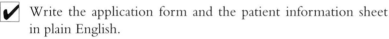

Pitfall	Solution
Application form not completed properly	Follow instructions very carefully and answer all the questions, even if not applicable

Protocol not written clearly	Ensure that the protocol is detailed and is very clear what you plan to do
Badly written patient information sheet	Make sure that you do not use jargon Use plain English Make sure that you address all potential questions
Access to the subject group not clear	Gain permission from the relevant consultant, senior nurse for research/DNO, senior nurse for the relevant unit
Confidentiality can be breached	Ensure that no names appear on data sheets, tapes, etc. Use codes instead
There is a risk to the patient's health	Do not contemplate a research study that has the potential to affect a patient's health adversely. This will not get approval

REFERENCES

CERES (1991) *Bulletin of Medical Ethics* **67**: 4.

Clinical Resources and Audit Group (1993) Cited in University of Dundee (1994) *Moving to Audit: What Every Nurse, Midwife and Health Visitor Needs to Know About Professional Audit.* Scotland: University of Dundee.

Declaration of Helsinki (1989) *Recommendations Guiding Physicians in Biomedical Research involving Human Subjects.* World Medical Association.

Department of Health (1991) *Local Research Ethics Committees.* HSG (91)5, August.

Department of Health (1997) *Ethics Committees' Review of Multicentre Research: Establishment of Multicentre Research Ethics Committees.* HSG (97)23, May.

Department of Health (2001) *Research Governance Framework for Health and Social Care* (Draft). Consultation paper. Available from http//www.doh.gov.uk/research/announcements/researchgovernanceconsult.htm.

Frankena, W.K. (1963) Cited in Seedhouse, D. (1998) *Ethics – The Heart of Health Care,* 2nd edition. Chichester: Wiley, p. 136.

Gillon, R. (1986) *Philosophical Medical Ethics.* Chichester: Wiley.

Human Rights Act (1998) London: HMSO.

ICH Harmonised Tripartate Guideline for Good Clinical Practice for Research (1996) Cited in Medical Research Council (1998) *Guidelines for Good Clinical Practice in Clinical Trials.* London: MRC

Neuberger, J. (1992) *Ethics and Health Care: The Role of Research Ethics Committees in the United Kingdom.* London: King's Fund Institute.

NHS Executive (1998) *A First Class Service: Quality in the New NHS.* London: HMSO.

ETHICAL ISSUES

UKCC (1987) *Confidentiality: An Elaboration of Clause 9 of the Second Edition of the UKCC's Code of Professional Conduct for the Nurse, Midwife and Health Visitor.* London: UKCC.

UKCC (1989) *Exercising Accountability: A Framework to Assist Nurses, Midwifes and Health Visitors to Consider Ethical Aspects of Professional Practice.* London: UKCC.

UKCC (1992) *Code of Professional Conduct for the Nurse, Midwife and Health Visitor.* London: UKCC.

UKCC (1996) *Guidelines for Professional Practice.* London: UKCC.

9

VENTURING INTO THE FIELD

Maggie Tarling and Linda Crofts

- Gaining access
- Consent
- Lack of subjects
- Ensuring efficient data collection
- Staying sane

INTRODUCTION

You may appreciate by now that planning a research project is very time-consuming. A lot of work has to be invested in preparing a research study before you actually get to the stage of collecting data in the field. One of the first major obstacles to overcome is gaining access to the area you are interested in. When trying to gain access you will find that there are important individuals in positions of power who can dictate your access to staff, resources and patients and can severely limit your ability to conduct your study. There is still an attitude of paternalism within the NHS and you may find that both medical and nursing staff seem to feel that they know what is best for their patients and take a very protective role in restricting researchers' access to them.

If your research involves patients then many local ethics committees insist that a medical consultant must take responsibility for a research project. No matter how unfair this may seem, when many doctors are often totally unaware of nursing issues, it is very much to your advantage to work with medical staff if for no other reason than they can place serious obstacles in your way later on if you fail to consult with them. Therefore you will need to ask the appropriate consultant for permission to approach his or her patients. It is only courtesy to do this in any case, especially if medical teams are themselves conducting research, as it is important that your own research does not clash, and because patients are advised only to take part in one research study at a time. However, the main problem with involving medical staff in your research is their lack of understanding about nursing research, particularly if it is using qualitative methodology.

'Explaining the research area to those taking part was difficult especially those from a different professional background who seemed to find the concepts of a more qualitative approach difficult to grasp.'

Alison Hill

Indeed, even if your research is quantitative in design, if the research hypothesis runs contrary to established medical beliefs then it is often difficult if not impossible to gain access. Nursing staff can be equally difficult if your research is at all controversial. In order to overcome the major obstacle of gaining access, the researcher needs to become politically aware and sensitive to these issues. Gaining the cooperation of key staff will ensure that the process of collecting your data is as smooth as possible.

'There was a surprising resistance from the consultant in charge of the area. The approach was not a qualitative one, but as the hypothesis ran contrary to accepted understanding he was not convinced about the value of the research. Such was the resistance that it was decided to approach another area. Subsequent research has supported our original views.'

Maggie Tarling

There are many other potential problems that can await you in the field. Box 9.1 outlines some of the more common ones.

Box 9.1 *Common problems*

- You cannot find sufficient numbers of subjects for your study.
- You find that the resources that you will need to carry out your study are not available to you.
- The equipment you need to use does not work.
- The staff do not have time or the motivation to help you.
- You are rapidly running out of time to complete your data collection.

VENTURING INTO THE FIELD

Remember that no matter what provisions you make, you should always expect the unexpected. Careful planning in advance can make your life as a researcher a lot easier.

MAJOR OBSTACLES TO COLLECTING YOUR DATA

Gaining access

The first problem you should consider is that of getting access to your subjects, whether this is in a hospital or community setting. Subjects is a rather impersonal term for the group of people who will form your sample group(s). They may be patients, carers, members of staff or members of the public. Whoever your subjects are, the same considerations for access apply and this is not easy in some cases. You should ask yourself the following questions before you start:

 Who do you need to talk to about getting access to the clinical area?

 Will you be allowed to approach patients/subjects?

Will What facilities will you need in the clinical area, such as a room for interviews, a power point to run equipment, a telephone, etc.?

 Will these facilities be available to you when you need them?

What will the staff feel about someone coming in from outside the area to do research?

 How will staff feel about someone from within the area taking on a researcher's role?

 Can you expect cooperation from relevant staff?

How many subjects who fit your criteria can you expect to come in contact with within the time limit that you have?

The most effective way to answer these questions is actually to visit the clinical area that you are interested in and to talk to the relevant staff. If you are not familiar with the area then you will have to approach the relevant senior member of nursing staff in the first instance. This individual is useful to talk to because they will be aware of local conditions and the most relevant local people to approach. Getting the support of senior staff can make your life much easier in gaining support from more junior staff within the clinical area.

If you wish to carry out your research in an entirely different hospital then you are best advised to write to the Director of Nursing seeking permission before negotiating access any further. If the hospital has a senior nurse for research then arrange to meet at the earliest opportunity to get advice on local issues and to pave the way for you in terms of accessing your field.

It is very important to have a clear protocol written in order to help explain exactly what you propose to do. Some individuals may also insist on ethical approval before you speak to them about a particular research project. This can be a bit of a catch-22 because there may be times when you need to talk to clinical staff directly about certain issues before you make your ethics committee application, such as making a realistic estimate of the numbers of subjects that will be available for your study and how long you think it will take to conduct the data collection. When you do meet staff you will have to convince them of the following:

- ✔ Your research is ethical and you have Local Research Ethics Committee (LREC) approval for the study.
- ✔ Your research is relevant.
- ✔ You have thought through the protocol very carefully.
- ✔ You will not disrupt the work routine unduly.
- ✔ You will not disrupt individual patient care.
- ✔ You are open to suggestions from clinical staff.
- ✔ You are sympathetic to the problems that staff may have.

This process takes time and you should make allowances for this. All clinical staff are very busy and you may find delays in talking to people because of their workload. You need to give yourself at least a month for paving the way in getting access to the relevant clinical area. And always remember that you need to give extra time for multicentre studies where several areas will have to be approached.

The process can be quite stressful for the researcher. Up till now your research would have been evaluated by colleges, your supervisor and financial or ethical committees. Approaching clinical staff can be quite different where your work will be given a critical evaluation that somehow seems more personal. You may encounter problems if your research appears to contradict the prevailing ideas within the clinical setting. This can be particularly difficult and is where you need to be confident in your research idea and have an in-depth understanding of the issues around your particular area. You will need to develop good communication skills. You should also believe in your own research to be able to convince others that your research is worth doing.

Threats to the culture

Extract from the researcher's diary: 'Eros' – a study of the social construction of male sexuality in the field of GU practice

The first hurdle was to secure access to my first choice sites. There are two clinics on sites which are less than two miles apart, but very different in their population profile, throughput, numbers of staff and extent of research activity. Both clinics, however, are managed within the same directorate, the head of which undertook to present my project to his consultants, and the decision about whether or not access would be given to each of their clinics would be theirs. I was subsequently invited to meet them, together with a clinical psychologist. No other member of their teams was present. The outcome was that access would be given at the smaller clinic, but not at the larger of the two. My impression from this interview, and other sources, was that:

- *I was told in advance of submitting the proposal to the ethics committee that the subject matter and methodology were contentious and unlikely to be passed without powerful support(ers).*

- *Access to one of the clinical arenas was not granted by one of the consultants, as they were 'too busy' and could not accommodate the extra work ... even though it would not require the staff in the clinic to conduct interviews or briefing of clients.*

One of the gatekeeper consultants was worried that the interviews might be so disturbing that they would trigger off 'psychiatric episodes' in clients and it would be the doctors who would have to 'sort them out'. Although some would agree that men are so insecure in their sexual identities that any exploration of their sexuality would initiate emotional trauma,

(Continued)

in this case the message would appear rather to expose the patriarchal and proprietorial attitude of doctors towards their patients. It also appears to reinforce the experience and suspicion of many nurses, for instance, that clinical research which does not conform to the positivist, biomedical paradigm is regarded with suspicion if not hostility by some doctors. Talking with patients appears to be more problematic and 'invasive' than randomised controlled drug trials and new or experimental surgical interventions!

Anthony Pryce

Nurses researching nurses

So far we have mainly considered the issues of gaining access to the field when the focus of your research is patients. However, many nursing research projects focus on nurses, i.e. nurses' attitudes to … , nurses' knowledge of … , the experiences of nurses working with … , as well as studies addressing the organisation of care and professional development issues. If you are a nurse researcher who has nurses as a subject group then there are some important issues you will need to address before you begin collecting your data.

As a nurse researcher working in the field you have a responsibility to ensure that the nurses you wish to participate in the research feel involved and have some ownership of the study. If you are using qualitative methodology then this statement is consistent with qualitative philosophical values. You will already be well aware that you are not seeking objectivity in your study but credibility (Sandelowski, 1986) and that you need to invest considerable time and effort in your subject group in return for their cooperation. There has been some criticism of the way in which traditional researchers have entered the field, 'grabbed' their data and left, referred to by Anne Oakley as 'smash and grab' (Oakley, 1981). Le Roux (1988) also identified that frequently when research was being carried out on the ward by a clinical researcher, the nurses did not see it as anything to do with them.

If you are planning to carry out an observational study involving nurses in an area where you are not known you will need to spend time getting to know the staff and the culture before you are able to start your data collection. This can involve anything from attending meetings to working alongside the staff for full shifts as a practising nurse (for which you are likely to need an honorary contract if you are not employed by that hospital or community setting). However,

VENTURING INTO THE FIELD

while this may be reasonable if you are a full-time PhD student, for a part-time degree student who has less than a year to complete the study this scenario is clearly too time-consuming. Consequently, many part-time researchers choose to conduct their study either in their own practice setting or, if they are a lecturer, in one in which they already have an established relationship.

While there are obvious advantages in carrying out research in your own field it is also fraught with problems as described by Field (1991), who advises against it, and James (1984) who used to make outrageous remarks to remind staff in unguarded moments that there was a researcher in their midst. While you have the advantage of already knowing the field there are a number of issues that you will need to consider:

 How to make clear to staff which is your research role and which is your 'normal' role.

 Consider whether you need to separate out fieldnotes.

 How do you feed back unfavourable findings to the staff?

How do you deal with the problem of witnessing poor practice?

If you are a lecturer, a manager or perhaps a clinical nurse specialist, the staff need to know in what capacity you are working in their practice setting. The boundaries are even more blurred if you are the ward sister researching practice in your own ward. It is virtually impossible, for example, to be working alongside a student nurse for a shift and not observe other things going on which you wish to write up in your fieldnotes. Equally it is difficult to be working on the unit on a research day yet not get involved in an issue which pertains to your 'other' job. In the case of participant observation what is particularly problematic is when, as a researcher, you witness poor or unsafe nursing practice. In the case of action research the boundaries are impossible to test out as the research revolves around problem-solving cycles in practice.

One solution to these issues is to be absolutely explicit in the written information you give to participants when asking for their consent to take part in the study. You should ensure that participants know that your fieldnotes will reflect observations made in the set-ting whether you are there in your work capacity or as a researcher for a fixed period of time, given how impossible it is to tease out one from the other. You should also make explicit that if you witness poor or unsafe practice then as a registered nurse you have a professional responsibility under the UKCC Code of Conduct to report it.

However, you should ensure that when you are carrying out tape-recorded interviews then these are as a researcher and that information is confidential and anonymous. Failure to emphasise this will inevitably mean that participants will self-censor what they are prepared to say to you. You might want to think about carrying out interviews at times of the day or evening when you would not normally be around in your 'work' role.

You can also find that the issue of poor practice crops up during interviews. All researchers experience the dilemma of whether to include data that come out once the tape recorder is switched off and this is a matter for your own conscience, depending on the nature of the material. However, in one case where a researcher was discussing a practice issue during a taped interview, it became clear that the participant had a very poor basic knowledge of the subject and was clearly giving inappropriate care to her client group. The researcher had no option but to turn off the tape, put the interview to one side and talk about the practice issue.

There is always a problem with how to share less than complimentary findings with the staff group. Whether you have interviewed staff, patients or both, the reflexive nature of the joint ownership of qualitative research means that you cannot just abandon your field when your data collection is complete; you need to arrange in advance when and how you will discuss your findings. Again this is best addressed before you start the study. By warning staff that the results may not be favourable, and asking them whether they would like you to discuss the results with them, however they turn out, you have at least prepared yourself and them for what may lie ahead.

Consent

Getting consent from patients is the next important issue that can be a major problem for a researcher. Consent must be sought for all forms of research. Many LRECs insist on written consent for all research, including surveys, questionnaires or interviews. As stated in Chapter 8 it is important that a patient's right to refuse to participate is protected. The process of consent is therefore very important and very difficult. This is a potential minefield for researchers when they go into the field to start to collect data for their research. It is imperative that the patient is not coerced into participating. This is where the dilemma lies for a researcher. You have a need to conduct the research, therefore patients or their relatives need to be approached, but this can be very difficult when the research may be very sensitive and may have the potential to upset an individual. Some LRECs insist on a witness being present and signing the consent form as well to ensure that there is no undue pressure put upon patients or their relatives.

It is just as important to gain written consent from nurses and other health professionals taking part in research as they should be afforded the same rights of confidentiality, information and the option to withdraw from the study without it affecting their employment. As already indicated, you can actually save yourself a lot of problems in the long run by being absolutely explicit in the information sheet about the issues involving participant observation in particular.

'In my experience of approaching patients for consent to participate in research patients tend to respond in one of three ways. There are those who are happy to participate and feel that they want to give something back for the help and treatment that they receive. These individuals tend to respond very positively very quickly. Then there are those who for whatever reason want nothing to do with research and refuse very quickly. These two types of responses are very easy to deal with. The group that can be problematic are those who sort of feel that they ought to. So they say yes but they don't really want to participate. This is difficult because you have a dilemma; you need to approach patients and you often have a deadline to meet, so you need patients to consent but equally you do not want to have patients feeling coerced into consenting. You should give patients plenty of opportunity to withdraw if they so wish, without making them feel bad about it.'

Maggie Tarling

Whatever careful consideration has been given to a research protocol, there may be great problems getting consent from patients once you get into the clinical area. The ethical process is very much driven by the patient, who has the right to refuse to participate. You should not assume that just because an ethics committee has passed your study as ethical patients will consent to participate. In general, research that is non-threatening will have a better chance of finding consenting patients than more invasive protocols. This not only includes research that may be physically invasive, but also research that may be personally invasive or very time-consuming. This does not mean that more complex studies should not be attempted but one must expect them to take longer to complete. If lack of consent from patients becomes a major problem then the research protocol may have to be re-evaluated.

If your research involves nurses as subjects the time-consuming nature of a study is also an issue. Participant observation does not necessarily involve extra time on the nurse's part, but interviews and questionnaires certainly do. Although the senior nurse may have given you blanket permission to access the field and the ethics committee may have given approval, individual nurses may quite reasonably decide that they do not have time to participate. It is up to you as a researcher to bend over backwards to meet the nurses on their own terms if you want to get your data, for example by coming in at the weekend when the ward may be quieter and by making the return of questionnaires as easy as possible.

Lack of numbers

Insufficient numbers of subjects being recruited is a common problem and causes many a research study to bite the dust. Such a major problem requires careful consideration at the planning stage. You will also need to take account of holidays and seasonal changes. The summer holidays period, for example, can be a problem because both medical staff and patients may be away. Some areas may also be involved with clinical exams, which means that routine work is suspended during this time. You will need to find out about these events and plan your data collection around them.

Some research studies are definitely seasonal. We recently planned a major two-year study evaluating the role of a key worker using an integrated care pathway for patients who had sustained a fractured neck of femur. By the time we had the proposal agreed, the funding secured and the key worker in post it was April and we would have to wait until the autumn to get sufficient numbers of patients in again.

'I have found that practitioners of every description suffer what I term the "optimistic heuristic". That is they overestimate the amount of work they actually do. When investigating how many patients will be available to you who fit your criteria it is important not to depend upon estimates. If it is at all possible then you should get access to actual audit figures of work done. This will be more accurate. Though of course the figures may not reflect the work that will be done.'

Maggie Tarling

If you find that there will not be sufficient numbers of patients available to you then a re-evaluation of the study protocol may be required. If you cannot change the protocol then you may have to plan more time for the data collection. If time is a problem then you may have to investigate the possibility of using other areas, but you need to consider having to make further ethics committee applications if sites are outside your area.

DATA COLLECTION

Once you finally get out there to collect the data it is important to ensure that your data collection is accurate. You only get one shot at this. It is therefore of great importance to ensure that you collect the important data. It is extremely difficult to go back over records or rely on memory in order to collect data you missed as important retrospectively. This also has the potential of introducing bias into your results unless your study was actually designed like this in the beginning. Records should be taken at the time.

The role of the pilot study

The aim of the pilot study is to identify potential problems with your study design. The pilot study may seem time-consuming, especially when you have a tight schedule, but it is well worth doing. In fact it will save you time in the long term. You aim to run your protocol, interview schedule, etc., with a small number of subjects to evaluate how well your research tools will perform. The pilot will also help to identify any potential practical problems that may arise once you get going. Often these problems are not apparent until you start and it is important to identify them as early as possible. You must remember that you will still need LREC approval to conduct a pilot study and you will have to return to the LREC to make changes to the protocol if you find you need to change it.

A pilot study will:

 Ensure that all equipment, questionnaires, etc., work effectively and reliably.

 Identify specific problems that subjects may have with the protocol; for example:

- Will the study take up too much time?
- Are questions open to misinterpretation?
- Are subjects comfortable with the data collection technique?
- Are the facilities available appropriate, e.g. give enough privacy?

 Indicate any problems with the data:

- Will the data be easy to analyse?
- Is the data easy to encode?
- Are audiotapes understandable?

 Indicate whether you are collecting all the relevant data.

'Carrying out my pilot study for interviews was just so essential because it was pretty much a disaster! I had tested the recording equipment in advance as per guidance from countless experienced research authors. I also tested on the day in the interview room. My mistake was that I tested the tape recorder on myself. My first interviewee turned out to have a touch of laryngitis, we had a wonderful interview and when I excitedly went home to transcribe it I could hardly hear her. It took hours to transcribe with the volume turned up fully.'

Patricia Fathers

'It was important to be confident about equipment. I had a small camcorder. On one occasion it did not work and I had to do the whole interview over again.'

Alison Hill

Interviews

Some reference has already been made to the possible pitfalls of conducting interviews. All good research books will talk about the importance of testing all your equipment and finding a quiet room where you are undisturbed. The reality is quite different for very practical reasons. First, if you are conducting interviews on a hospital ward or in a health centre, space is at a premium and you may have to resort to using Sister's office, thus inconveniencing other members of staff. If you are interviewing members of staff in work time it is quite possible that they will be bleeped or called away to deal with a crisis despite efforts to let everyone know they are not available. The room itself may have insufficient chairs or no electrical socket to run your tape recorder from.

Basically you are just going to have to do the best you can. One researcher resorted to a large microphone during tape recording which she explained was because many of her interviews had been conducted in a hospital next to a major rail terminal and therefore the dialogue had been punctuated with rail announcements and trains leaving and arriving. In our own hospital, conversations are frequently interrupted by the helicopter taking off and landing. It is important to know how your equipment works and to be able to adjust the recording level appropriately.

> 'My second mistake lay with the venue selection for the interviews. I had allowed myself to be organised by the enthusiastic and willing clinical staff. The room commandeered for the occasion was an office which was accessed from another. Large notices on the door did not stop a stream of interruptions. The interview recordings were punctuated with a series of crashes (the door opening), additional voices (sorry I didn't realise the room was engaged, do you know where xxxxx is?) and thuds (the door closing again). I should have been much more involved and assertive with selecting and securing a suitable area and indeed I remedied this for the main study.'
>
> *Patricia Fathers*

Sometimes you might be conducting interviews in someone's home. While this has the advantage of the participant being at ease in their own surroundings, it makes you the guest who can be asked to leave. You may feel that you have to think twice about asking difficult questions or ones that may upset the participant. Worse still,

VENTURING INTO THE FIELD

if you do upset your respondent you are honour bound to remain after the interview until you feel they have sufficiently recovered. A number of researchers have talked about the experience of leaving someone's home very shaken by what they have heard or feeling guilty about the emotions they have raised (Finch, 1984; Flately, 1993). This indicates that it may be as well to suggest that there is someone with the participant once you have gone if you are asking particularly sensitive questions, e.g. about bereavement. It would also be sensible to make use of your own support network for yourself. Remember that while the participant may feel fine ten minutes after you have gone, you may feel awful for a long time.

If you are conducting semi-structured interviews you may find your participants are either more than willing to chat, often spanning more than one question, frequently digressing but nevertheless providing plenty of data, or they respond with yes or no answers and it is up to you to probe, encourage and engage them in the topic. Sometimes very guarded answers may be because you have not put the participant sufficiently at ease and indeed the main data come out after the tape has been switched off and they are about to leave. However, it may genuinely be because they do not feel they have very much to say. Having said that, some of the more thoughtful responses can provide the richest data.

You may encounter a situation where you become aware that the participant is basically not telling the truth or that the response is entirely contradictory to what happened in practice. For example, in one series of interviews a colleague was conducting, a ward manager clearly stated that all the nurses had been involved in creating the ward philosophy when all the other respondents said they had never seen it. While this may be very perplexing at the time, do bear in mind that all qualitative data has potential and indeed may qualify some of your notes from participant observation.

If you are attempting theoretical sampling and conducting a series of unstructured interviews then you run the very real risk of your participants saying absolutely nothing. Conducting unstructured interviews is highly skilled and not to be recommended to the first-time researcher. The best advice is to shadow someone who is conducting this type of research and learn from them before doing it alone.

Questionnaires

If you are using an 'off the shelf' questionnaire then you need to get permission from the author to use it. You should also make quite sure that it is suitable for its intended use. For example, the Beck Depression Inventory (1962) was intended to measure states of depression yet it is frequently thrown in as an extra in studies looking at stress, anxiety, breaking bad news and so forth.

If you are using your own questionnaire then it needs to be piloted to test it for validity. Even before the pilot it is a good idea to ask a colleague to look over it to point out obvious ambiguities. There are three validities to questionnaires:

- Face validity i.e. what it looks like
- Content validity – the form the questions take
- Construct validity – what the problem focus is.

You need to address all these to your specific sample group if you are to get a significant return rate. The list below outlines the features of a good questionnaire.

 If the questionnaire is lengthy there should be justification for it.

 If it is too short respondents will question its worthwhileness.

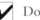 Do not try and cram in too many issues.

 Value people's time; make it brief and to the point (ease of use).

 Design it for your specific target group.

 Offer feedback or some interaction as a reward.

 Offer yourself in the introduction as a credible source for doing the survey.

 Guarantee confidentiality and anonymity.

 Give a clear exposition of purpose.

Use blocking, i.e. arrange content in 'blocks' of topics.

Beware of status questions – it is very easy to imply value ordering for married/single, employed/unemployed, etc.

Asking for date of birth is better than asking for age ranges.

 The biggest challenge is getting your questionnaires returned to you. First class stamped addressed envelopes are considered the best option because they label the study as important, but this is obviously costly. Many nurses use internal mail systems which are less than reliable and you would need to ask permission to use it. Asking people to complete questionnaires while you are present has the obvious advantage of getting a good response rate but could be viewed as coercive. It is very unusual to get more than a 70% return rate for a postal questionnaire, so you need to allow for this in your sample size, particularly if you want to do a statistical analysis.

Keeping records

It is important to keep accurate records. To comply with the confidentiality of patients or staff this information *must not* be kept with the actual data and an individual must not be identifiable from the data sheets themselves. However, there may be a need to look back, at a later date, on details of patients who have participated in research if there is a query about any adverse event that occurs later. You may then keep a separate secure record of subjects' details in order to be able to track details back to a particular subject. However, it is of paramount importance that you comply with the Data Protection Act (1998) to ensure that you protect the rights of subjects. It is also very important to be careful when you are dealing with data that will be transferred to another party electronically. You must be sure that the transfer is secure and that you are not transferring sensitive information. It is important to note that data sent outside the NHS net is not secure unless steps are taken to encrypt it.

If you are conducting taped interviews you must ensure that the name does not appear on any of the tape recordings or subsequent transcripts. It is up to you to devise a coding system that ensures you know the identity but no one else does.

Data sheets

Data sheets are a convenient way of recording data so as to make analysis easier at a later date. Table 9.1 shows an example of part of a data sheet. Recording empirical data in this way can be useful for analysing the data later.

Table 9.1 *An example of a data sheet*

Subject number	Age	State anxiety	Diagnosis of cancer	Stress score
1	35	60	0	27
2	61	30	1	18
3	70	44	1	33

Some data are quite easy to record, as the values are self-evident, such as age. But you may be collecting information that is more difficult to convert into numerical values. In this situation you can code the information to produce a number. In the example shown in Table 9.1, a diagnosis of cancer was recorded for these individuals. For those with a diagnosis a code of 1 was given and for those without a diagnosis of cancer a code of 0 was given. This enables a more straightforward analysis of data, but it is limited and this sort of information has to be treated very carefully. It would be meaningless to calculate a mean value for diagnosis, for example. It would be more sensible to calculate and talk about the percentages of those patients with and without a diagnosis of cancer. This sort of coding may be useful for analysis but it loses the richness of experience. For example, you cannot tell anything about the feelings of these individuals about their diagnosis or the impact that this may have on an individual. Data sheets can be very useful in keeping your records clearly and enabling easier analysis, but one must consider the type of information and the appropriateness of the way it is recorded.

If you are conducting a qualitative study then you will need to transcribe your tapes as soon as possible. If you do this yourself then you have the benefit of reliving every bit of the interview and can begin to form some impressions as to its significance, but it is also extraordinarily time-consuming. You also feel obliged to transcribe verbatim which means you pick up every hesitation, repetition and shuffle which later on you will almost certainly discard. It can easily take eight hours to transcribe one hour's worth of interview, so if you do not feel this is a good use of your time either get an experienced audio typist to do it for you (for which you will have to pay) or, if the interviews are supplementary to your main data collection, make a summary of them. Transcripts should be double-spaced with a wide margin on both sides of the page to facilitate coding in the analysis stage.

'On listening to the first two tapes I realised that to transcribe verbatim would be very time consuming and would not add anything to the data. I therefore wrote a summary of each interview with quotes where it seemed appropriate. The interviews were fifty minutes in length and it usually took three hours to summarise each tape.'

Alison Hill

It is when you come to transcribe your tapes that you realise what you have omitted to ask and you cannot go back.

> '*I planned to conduct interviews as part of my data collection. No problem I thought, these people know me and I know them (I'd been the link teacher there for nearly two years). What I completely forgot to collate, however, was biographical details until well after I'd finished the interviews. It was hopeless, I only had a vague knowledge of how long they had each been in practice, I couldn't remember accurately who had specialist qualifications and who hadn't. When it came to transcribing the interviews and identifying themes within the practice carried out, the significance of who had what professional education and training in the past became all too clear.*'
>
> Patricia Fathers

Monitoring

It is important to keep monitoring and evaluating the progress of data collection. This process should identify any problem early. If this is done on a regular basis then problems can be identified early on in the process and can be remedied without any major harm to the research study. You only have one chance of collecting data. You cannot go back and recapture that individual's experience.

> '*It was only at the end of the study that I realised that my sample group was flawed. It was an ethnographic study and two nurses had dropped out of the interviews and I replaced them with two others. It was only during the data analysis I realised that both nurses who dropped out had been black SENs, leaving a predominantly white SRN sample group despite the predominance of black SENs on the ward. It was too late to do anything about it.*'
>
> Linda Crofts

Getting others to collect data

You may be in a position to have a research assistant to collect data for you. If so, you must allow a lot of time for briefing your assistant to make sure that they understand exactly what is required. The importance of following the protocol cannot be stressed enough. The structure of questions, how tests should be carried out, what observations are recorded and how they are recorded are important issues that must be addressed. An assistant must be given training and close supervision.

If you have someone working with you, it is important to ensure that individual bias in collecting data does not enter the data. Both researchers need to make sure that data are collected in the same way and protocols must be very explicit and spell out exactly what steps should be taken. In an empirical study technique becomes important when using interview techniques or assessments which may not be totally objective. One way of ensuring that different observers are rating in the same way is to ensure that the same observations made by different observers correlate closely. This is known as inter-rater reliability.

The worst position to be in is to be reliant upon staff within a clinical area to collect data for you. If this situation is approached carefully it can be controllable, but there are many pitfalls. In general, research has a low priority in the ordinary run of things. Clinical staff have a job to do and are not there for your convenience; the data collection may distract from their duty to provide care to patients; they may also be too busy to collect data for you. Therefore this way of approaching data collection is not recommended. However, if this is the only avenue open to you then you must make sure that staff understand exactly what is involved. It is best to keep things as simple as possible; if data collection fits the established routine then it is more likely to be done. It is a good idea to visit the area and talk to people directly. Providing incentives may also be useful, such as including individuals as authors of a paper, providing training opportunities to staff, letting staff with an interest in research get an opportunity to get hands-on experience of the research process. Always give feedback to staff when you have finished any research study. Staff are often neglected in this respect and they do appreciate being kept up to date with what is happening. Your relationship with clinical staff is important. Staff who have been encouraged and have been communicated with will be more cooperative and keen to participate in further research. You will also find them a source of support for yourself.

You may have a situation where you are asking patients to collect data for you. The most common format for this is the use of diaries. Patients are asked to record certain events or symptoms in a diary format whilst they are at home. This technique requires a very committed and motivated patient in order to be successful. This is not without its problems. Even the most dedicated individual may at times forget to make records. Therefore this sort of data can be unreliable. Electronic diaries available these days make data entry easy and more reliable. They can be programmed to collect the data and record the date and time that an entry is actually made, thus making the data collection more accurate. The data can easily be downloaded straight into a computer database, making analysis more straightforward. Though expensive, such electronic diaries can be very useful research tools when trying to access what happens to the progress of a patient within the community setting.

CONCLUSIONS; STAYING SANE

Staying sane during the research process is difficult at any time, but more so when data are being collected. This can be the most frustrating phase as despite all the careful planning and hard work up to this point so many things can go wrong. Problems that have not been anticipated can come to light at this stage and sometimes mean that a well-designed study in principle does not get off the ground in practice. Good communication is the key. Keep well informed as to what is happening in the area. Get to know staff and their point of view. This is very helpful in getting staff on your side. They can also be a source of help and support to you personally. It is also important for your own sanity to seek support from colleagues and to use a supervisor or mentor in helping you through difficulties. Above all else, remember that your sense of humour may be your biggest asset in helping you through the ups and downs of life as a researcher.

KEY POINTS

 Ensure that you have approached the most appropriate staff about getting permission to conduct the study.

 Visit the clinical area to see how the routine works and to assess how you will be able to fit into the routine without too much disruption.

 Ensure that you have accurate figures about the numbers of patients available to you who will fit your criteria.

VENTURING INTO THE FIELD

Ensure that you have spent time in the clinical area talking to staff about what you plan to do.

 Listen to clinical staff and their concerns and suggestions.

 Conduct a pilot study where appropriate.

✔ Be familiar with all the equipment that you will use.

✔ Be methodical about collecting and storing your data.

PITFALLS AND HOW TO AVOID THEM

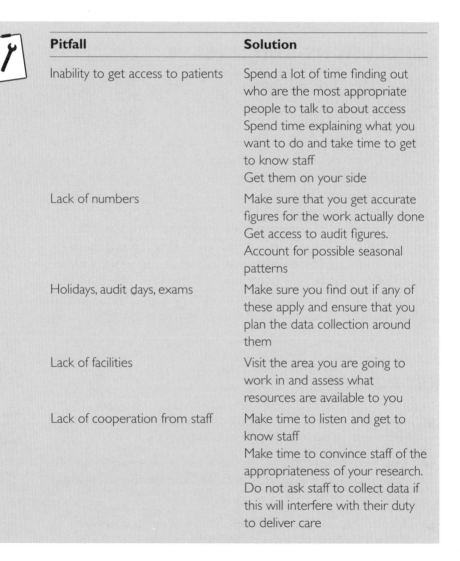

	Pitfall	Solution
	Inability to get access to patients	Spend a lot of time finding out who are the most appropriate people to talk to about access Spend time explaining what you want to do and take time to get to know staff Get them on your side
	Lack of numbers	Make sure that you get accurate figures for the work actually done Get access to audit figures. Account for possible seasonal patterns
	Holidays, audit days, exams	Make sure you find out if any of these apply and ensure that you plan the data collection around them
	Lack of facilities	Visit the area you are going to work in and assess what resources are available to you
	Lack of cooperation from staff	Make time to listen and get to know staff Make time to convince staff of the appropriateness of your research. Do not ask staff to collect data if this will interfere with their duty to deliver care

VENTURING INTO THE FIELD

Lack of consent	Re-evaluate your study protocol. Find out what it is about the study that patients are not keen on. Can this be changed?
Patients withdrawing from the study	Is there a particular aspect of the study that patients find particularly stressful or difficult? Try to make sure that patients are not just consenting because they feel they ought to
Running out of time	Can you get more time? Try and plan for sufficient time. Can you expand into a different area?
Unforeseen events	Not a lot you can do about this except keep your sense of humour.

REFERENCES

Data Protection Act (1998) London: HMSO.

Field, P.A. (1991) Doing fieldwork in your own culture. In: Morse, J.M. (ed.) *Qualitative Nursing Research*, 2nd edition. Newbury Park, CA: Sage.

Finch, J. (1984) It's great to have someone to talk to about the ethics and politics of interviewing women. In: Bell, C. and Roberts, H. (eds) *Social Researching, Politics, Problems and Practice*. London: Routledge & Kegan Paul.

Flately, M. (1993) Hospitalisation and discharge of stroke patients: the relatives' experience. In: Wilson-Barnett, J. and Macleod Clark, J. (eds) *Research in Health Promotion and Nursing*, Basingstoke: Macmillan.

James, N. (1984) A postscript to nursing. In: Bell, C. and Roberts, H. (eds) *Social Researching, Politics, Problems and Practice*. London: Routledge & Kegan Paul.

Le Roux, B. (1988) Conflict of interest. *Nursing Times* **84**(29): 32–33.

Oakley, A. (1981) Interviewing women, a contradiction in terms. In: Roberts, H. (ed.) *Doing Feminist Research*. London: Routledge.

Sandelowski, M. (1986) The problem of rigor in qualitative research. *Advances in Nursing Science* **8**(3): 27–37.

10

REPORTING RESULTS

Maggie Tarling and Linda Crofts

INTRODUCTION

This chapter outlines separately the problems you may encounter when carrying out quantitative and qualitative data analysis. As with some of the previous chapters, you will need to refer to standard research textbooks to understand the theory behind your analysis.

The aim of this chapter is to ease the actual process.

PART ONE: REPORTING QUANTITATIVE DATA

- Levels of measurement
- Descriptive statistics
- Measures of variance
- Parametric and non-parametric tests

This is a very quick guide to reporting the results of quantitative research. It will not show you how to calculate the statistical tests described here but there are many books which deal with these issues in more depth and you are well advised to consult one of them. There is also no substitute for the expert advice of a statistician or supervisor. It is imperative that these issues are considered at the planning stage as it is too late when you have collected all your data.

Quantitative methods generate numbers. Variables of interest are observed and measured and a number is given to them. It is always important to remember that the numbers or data never 'know where they come from'. You can almost prove anything with numbers. Therefore it is important always to consider what the numbers mean. It is vital to ensure that the statistical analysis you choose fits the type of data you have collected, otherwise the results will be nonsensical. For example, if you have collected data on whether a patient has a diagnosis of cancer or not, and you give a numerical value to this event such as

0 for no and 1 for yes, it would not make sense to calculate a mean value for the diagnosis of cancer: a mean value of 0.3 for a diagnosis of cancer would be meaningless, either you have the diagnosis or you do not. It would be more sensible to talk about percentages of patients with and without a diagnosis of cancer. Always consider the nature of the numbers in front of you. Where did they come from and what do they mean? This sort of error is easy to make and has the potential to make your results meaningless. However, there are simple steps to take which will make the likelihood of falling into these traps less likely.

The results section

There are accepted ways of writing up your results for quantitative data. The results section only describes the results of statistical analysis without comment. The discussion section is where you attribute meaning to the results and where you put your results into the context of your literature review. Generally speaking, you need to use summary statistics to describe the data you have collected and then go on to use inferential statistics to make generalisations about your results.

The first useful thing to do is to assess the type of data you have collected. This will give an indication of the type of statistics you can apply to your data. This is known, in 'statistics speak', as assessing the level of measurement. There are four levels and each one will give information about the data.

Nominal levels of measurement enable you to categorise responses to a named category. For example, you may ask subjects to give their marital status. They may then be categorised as, single, married, divorced, widowed, cohabiting. The important thing to remember about this sort of data is that it is mutually exclusive, one cannot be single and married at the same time.

Ordinal levels of measurement enable you to put the response into a rank order. The most common example of this is the use of visual analogue scales, where a response is marked along a scale. This is a common method of assessing pain, where subjects indicate their level of pain on a scale, from no pain to severe pain. The important point to consider with these types of scales is that the interval between the points may not be equal. For example, if you use a five-point visual analogue scale to assess pain (0 = no pain, 1 = mid pain, 2 = moderate pain, 3 = severe pain, 4 = worst pain imaginable) the intervals between a score of 2 and 3 and between a score of 3 and 4 may not be the same, as individuals rate pain differently. A mild pain for one person may be a severe pain for another.

Interval and ratio levels of measurements assume that the intervals between points on the scale are equal. The sorts of data that fall into

Table 10.1 *Some examples of the different levels of measurement*

Level of measurement	Example
Nominal	Demographic data, marital status, diagnosis categories, gender
Ordinal	Visual analogue scales, e.g. pain scales, anxiety scales, attitude scales
Interval/ratio	Age, time, temperature, height, number of infections

this level are age, time, temperature and height. If someone is 36 years of age, we know that another person aged 37 years of age is one year older. If a patient had to wait six months for an outpatient appointment and another had to wait a year, then we know that the second patient waited twice as long as the first. Interval and ratio scales provide us with more information.

All the different levels of measurement are useful, but they provide different amounts of information. Categorising your data into levels of measurement (Table 10.1) enables you to choose the type of statistic it is best to use.

Descriptive statistics

Descriptive statistics summarise the data you have collected. At the end of your data collection you will have collected a vast amount of data. When you put information onto a data sheet it will not make a lot of sense at first. Table 10.2 shows the raw scores from a study of pre-operative anxiety. Looking at this data it is difficult to make any sense of what is going on. The aim of descriptive statistics is to help sort out and make some sense of the mass of numbers in front of you.

There are two general ways of describing the data:

- Measuring the *central tendency* or average
- Measuring the *variability* or spread.

Measuring the central tendency

Measuring the central tendency (Table 10.3) or average gives you an indication of the 'typical' values of numbers in front of you. The average value plays an important role in inferential statistics. Calculating the average can enable you to compare different groups. If the average value in one group is very different from the average value

Table 10.2 Responses to pre-operative questionnaire

Subject number	Pre-operative state anxiety	Age	Previous experience[a]	Trait anxiety	Perceived stress	Operation[b]
1	23	39	1	37	25	1
2	34	30	1	29	10	2
3	66	25	2	63	25	2
4	40	33	1	52	19	2
5	52	33	2	30	9	2
6	49	26	2	44	26	2
7	63	40	1	31	33	2
8	33	27	1	34	15	2
9	50	47	1	49	17	1
10	42	38	0	50	26	1
11	29	44	2	36	13	1
12	23	43	0	33	18	1
13	52	30	0	34	10	2
14	35	35	1	32	10	2
15	36	28	1	29	14	2
16	41	32	2	39	18	1
17	72	46	2	31	21	1
18	50	40	2	49	31	3
19	40	66	2	51	34	3
20	33	51	1	33	19	3
21	21	33	1	60	22	1
22	44	43	2	41	29	2
23	36	59	1	52	13	1
24	20	35	1	29	7	1
25	23	38	1	31	5	2
26	47	60	1	52	17	2
27	31	31	1	33	11	3
28	46	39	2	51	10	1
29	34	34	1	23	9	1
30	35	28	1	47	5	1

[a]Previous experience codes: 0 = nil, 1 = positive, 2 = negative.
[b]Operation codes: 1 = major, 2 = intermediate, 3 = minor.

in another group then there may indeed be a difference due to the variables you have manipulated. Calculating an average enables an initial assessment of this difference to be made. However, there are different sorts of average to calculate. Which one is most applicable depends on the level of measurement.

Table 10.3 *Measures of central tendency and most appropriate level of measurement they apply to*

Measure of central tendency	Definition	Most appropriate level of measurement
Mode	The most frequent value in the raw data	Nominal
Median	The middle value of the ranked raw data	Ordinal
Mean	The average value calculated as the total number of scores divided by the number of scores	Interval/ratio

Table 10.4 *Measures of variance*

Measure of variance	Definition	Level of measurement
Range	The range of values covered by the scores	Ordinal
Inter-quartile range	The range of the middle half of the scores	Ordinal
Standard deviation	An average of the deviation of each score from the mean	Interval/ratio

Measures of variance

Once you have measured the average value it is useful to measure the spread of the data. If you plot a graph known as a histogram for your data you will see that not all the values are close to the average or mean value. You will most probably find for the majority of data that most of the values will be around the mean, but not all. You will also find that for some groups of data the values are very close to the mean and for others the values are more spread out. This spread is known as the variance. This statistic also plays a central role in inferential statistics.

There are several ways of measuring the variance, Table 10.4 lists the most common ones in use.

Once you have chosen the most appropriate summary statistic it is usual to present this in tabular form. Using tables or graphs is often the best way of presenting your results.

Table 10.5 *The mean and standard deviations for age, stress, pre-operative anxiety and trait anxiety for the group of gynaecological surgical patients*

Variable	Mean	SD
Age	38.4	10.29
Stress	17.37	8.34
Pre-operative state anxiety	40.0	13.11
Trait anxiety	40.2	10.6

Reporting the data from Table 10.2

In order to summarise the data in Table 10.2, it is important to understand what the measures mean and from whom they were taken. This was a study that looked at pre-operative levels of anxiety in a group of gynaecology patients the day before surgery. The measures of anxiety were made using a well-established anxiety inventory or questionnaire, not a visual analogue scale. The values on this scale range from 20 = no anxiety to 80 = high level of anxiety. The patients' previous experience was measured by asking patients about their previous experience and then giving a code to the response: a score of 0 =no previous experience, 1 = a positive experience, 2 = a negative experience. The types of operation were categorised into 1 = major abdominal surgery, 2 = laparoscopy, 3 = minor surgery. The measure of perceived stress was derived from a hospital stress rating scale by counting the number of events the patients encountered; this provides a score of 0 for no stressful events to a maximum of 50. The variables of age, pre-operative anxiety, trait anxiety and stress can be summarised using mean and standard deviations (SD) (Table 10.5). There may be some argument about the utility of using these statistics for variables such as those from an anxiety inventory, but this will not be discussed here. For variables such as type of operation and previous experience, which are nominal types of data, it would be inappropriate to calculate mean values. You could use the modal value; however, it is useful to give an indication of all the values that can be represented in a frequency table (Table 10.6) or pie chart (Figure 10.1).

Choosing a statistical test

Once you have described the data it may be appropriate to carry on to perform inferential statistics. These enable you to make generalisable statements about your results. There are three questions that

Table 10.6 *Frequency table of previous experience of hospital for the gynaecology patients*

	Frequency	Percentage	Cumulative percentage
Nil	3	10.0	10.0
Positive experience	17	56.7	66.7
Negative experience	10	33.3	100.0
Total	30	100	

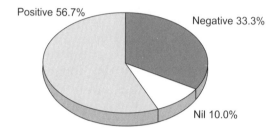

Fig. 10.1 *Previous experience of hospital. Data from Table 10.6 presented as a pie chart*

need to be considered when deciding which test to use on the data:

1 *Research design* – Have you looked at differences between groups or categories or have you looked at relationships between variables?

2 *Level of measurement* – Which level of measurement have you used?

3 *Variance* – Have the samples of data equal variances or homogeneity of variance?

There are two categories of inferential statistical tests: parametric and non-parametric tests.

Parametric tests use the raw scores in their calculation. They are carried out on data that are of interval/ratio level of measurement. But there are certain assumptions underlying the use of parametric tests: it is assumed that the data has a normal distribution and has a homogeneity of variance. A normal distribution has a symmetrical shape, with most of the values falling within the middle part of the curve and with extreme scores tailing off fairly rapidly on either side of the central area. Many variables in nature have this characteristic shape. This is taken advantage of in the calculation of inferential statistics.

Non-parametric tests are calculated on the ranks of the scores, not on the raw data. These tests are useful for ordinal levels of measurement or where the assumptions for the use of parametric tests do not hold.

Table 10.7 gives a quick reference guide to choosing a statistical test for some of the most common research designs. It is by no means comprehensive.

Table 10.7 *Common statistical tests and research designs*

	Investigating differences between groups					Investigating relationships between variables	Investigating differences between categories
	Two experimental conditions		Three or more experimental conditions				
	Related	Independent	Related	Independent		Correlation	
Parametric tests	Related *t*-test	Independent *t*-test	Related one-way ANOVA	Independent one-way ANOVA		Pearson	
Non-parametric tests	Wilcoxon	Mann–Whitney	Friedman	Kruskal-Wallis		Spearman	Chi-square

Related research designs have the same subjects responding to all the experimental conditions. Independent designs have different subjects in each experimental condition.

p-values

When you have calculated your inferential statistic you will have what is known as a *p*-value. It is important to note that the *p* stands for probability. What the *p*-value tells you is the probability that the results of your research occurred by chance and not by the manipulation of the research variables.

When talking about *p*-values you need to understand the notion of probability. Probability is measured from 1 to 0. An event with a probability of 0 is impossible and an event with a probability of 1 is inevitable (Figure 10.2). Most events lie somewhere between these two probabilities. You need to be fairly certain that the results of your research have not occurred by chance, so a level of significance is determined. The level of significance is determined by convention. This means the significance level is set at less than or equal to 0.05. If one thinks back to how probability is measured this gives a probability of 5 times in 100 of occurring by chance. If you want to have a stricter criterion, that is you want to be even more sure that your results have not occurred by chance, then you set the significance level at 0.01, that is a 1 in 100 chance of having occurred by chance. In order to determine if the results of your statistical analysis are statistically significant the *p*-value is compared to the level of significance. If it is less than or equal to the significance level, i.e. 0.05 or 0.01, then the results are deemed to be statistically significant.

When you assess the results of empirical research you must always remember that the results are measured in probabilities. The *p*-value

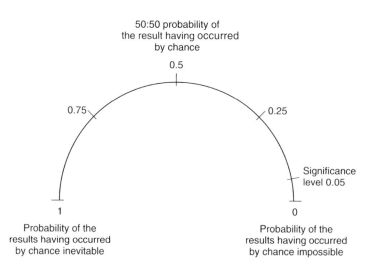

Fig. 10.2 *If the probability of the statistical analysis falls above the 0.05 significance level then the results are assumed to have occurred by chance. If it falls below the 0.05 level, i.e. nearer to 0, the results are assumed to be not due to chance, and are considered statistically significant*

gives an indication that the results could just have occurred by chance. The results are not set in stone and do not represent ultimate truth.

Statistical and clinical significance

As a last note it is important to consider the difference between statistical and clinical significance in research. Your research may have found a statistically significant difference between treatments or a relationship between variables. However, the difference may have been small. It is important to consider the impact that the results will have in the 'real world'. If you have compared the rate of urinary tract infection in patients receiving two different types of catheter, you may find that you have a statistically significant difference between the two groups. If that difference is small, for example a drop in infection rate of 1%, then the clinical significance of your results may not be very great. If, however, you find a large difference, for example a drop of 50% in infection rates, then the results will have a clinical significance, an impact on practice.

Though you may find a statistically significant result, it does not mean that the result has clinical significance. This is a problem with published results of research. Journals tend to publish the results of statistically significant research. However, it is often up to the reader to judge the clinical significance of the research. Reader beware.

When the numbers do not add up

Statistical analysis may seem straight forward and if data have been collected well and thought has been given to the research design and analysis there should be few problems. However, there are times when the numbers just do not seem to fit the statistical analysis. Or you may be facing a situation where the results seem bizarre and very difficult to interpret. Or your results are not statistically significant. Each situation has its own particular problems. This can be the most soul-destroying moment when you may feel that all your hard work has come to nothing. However, all is not lost and there are things you can do to improve the situation.

Was data collection accurate?

If the data seem strange or unexpected it is important to check that the data have been collected properly and errors have not been made. It is very easy to miss a decimal point, for example, and this can make all the difference. Outlying values are extreme values and present particular problems as they can have a profound influence upon statistical analysis.

The first step is to establish if the value is accurate and to ensure that an error has not been made. You have to be honest about this and not just assume an error has occurred and simply ignore the value. If you do exclude a value you must state this clearly in your analysis and the reasons why you have done this. You may have to accept an outlying value as genuine. There are statistical techniques available to control for this. I suggest if you do not have a good background in statistics that you approach a friendly statistician who will be able to help you.

You may be faced with a situation where you just cannot apply the statistical test you thought you would need. This sometimes happens when the underlying assumption of the statistical test has not been met. For example, many tests assume a normal distribution and your data may turn out to have a different distribution. This again is where a statistician will be able to advise you on another test.

What if your data are difficult to interpret?

Once you have analysed your data you may be faced with results that are totally unexpected or difficult to interpret. The results may run totally contrary to what you expected. To a certain extent this is much more interesting as it presents a challenge. 'Why?' is a researchers question and the art of research is to put the results of your research into context and to attempt to explain your results. Data that contradict your original hypothesis or a non-significant result do present a challenge. You may need to go back to the original literature and see if there is something that may have influenced your results. For example, is your population very different from previous studies? Was there a bias in your sampling method? Is the research environment very different? Are there factors that you have overlooked in your design or the way data were collected that may have influenced the results? A statistician may also be useful here in helping you to identify biases that may have contributed to the results.

All is not lost if you are faced with this situation. However, I would be underestimating the problem if I stated that this could easily be remedied. There is a bias in journals to only publish statistically significant studies. If you are looking to publish your results it can make the process much more difficult.

Beware the fishing trip

A 'fishing trip' occurs when numerous statistical tests are conducted with little rhyme or reason. This often happens when the researcher is unclear about the hypothesis in the first place and has given little thought to the type of analysis that will test the hypothesis. What happens then is that large amounts of often irrelevant data are collected and numerous statistical tests are carried out.

There are several problems with this approach. It is unethical to collect unnecessary data. It is a waste of subjects' time, effort and resources. As a researcher you have a responsibility to ensure that you utilise resources effectively. Collecting data 'just in case' is irresponsible. If you have given sufficient thought to the research design then this is unnecessary. The other major problem with this is that if you look hard enough, the odds are that you will find statistically significant results. This is meaningless if all you have done is manipulated the figures to get a significant result. Fishing trips are obvious to spot and reviewers and markers can easily distinguish between a well thought out study and one that is being analysed with the fishing rod.

KEY POINTS

☑ Always consider what statistical analysis to use at the planning stage.

☑ Always consider where the numbers have come from.

☑ Consider the level of measurement.

☑ Write the results section without comment.

☑ Use tables and graphs as much as possible.

PART TWO: REPORTING RESULTS FROM QUALITATIVE RESEARCH

- Keeping track of your data
- Immersing yourself in the data
- Coding transcripts
- Hearing what the data has to say
- Collapsing categories
- When the data do not fit…

There are few research textbooks that, when discussing qualitative research analysis, do not feel they have to discuss whether qualitative research is legitimate at all. This is because, apart from some notable

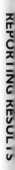

Box 10.1 *Parallel criteria of quantitative and qualitiative studies*

Quantitative	Qualitative
Internal validity	Credibility
External validity	Transferability
Reliability	Dependability
Objectivity	Confirmability

exceptions such as Polit and Hungler (1997), the majority of text-books continue to be written primarily in the quantitative paradigm with passing reference to qualitative research methods. Issues of tri-angulation, reliability, credibility and objectivity continue to be com-pared with traditional hallmarks of data analysis as though they are designed to measure the same thing, which they clearly do not. Guba and Lincoln (1989) summarised this point by showing that these terms form parallel criteria which are not interchangeable, as outlined in Box 10.1.

It is not the intention of this chapter to discuss the various merits of qualitative research or otherwise; this particular debate is alive and well in the academic journals. At the analysis stage it is important to recog-nise that qualitative research is interpretative and as such attempting to give quite different meaning to the data from quantitative research. The issues of validity and reliability are discussed in great detail in qualitative research textbooks such as Morse (1991) and in an excel-lent series of articles by Nolan and Behi (1995a, b, c) in the *British Journal of Nursing*. What this section does aim to do is give some guid-ance on managing and handling your data, which by this stage can be quite overwhelming.

It is worth mentioning here that not all research uses exclusively either quantitative or qualitative methodologies; many studies use a mixture of both, and this is certainly becoming very popular in health service research. For example, a study that wishes to focus on the care of a particular group of patients may use quantitative meth-ods to measure number of outpatient visits required, average waiting time, length of inpatient stay and any complications. However, it may also wish to conduct interviews with patients, their carers and key members of staff which would be analysed qualitatively. The dif-ferent methodologies here are designed to complement each other.

It is also very poor practice to use 'para' or 'quasi' statistics. These appear in reports in the form of 'most people said' ... 'a few people disagreed with the statement'. Either use statistics properly or do not use them at all.

Keeping track of your data

Reference has already been made in Chapter 9 to coding names for the purposes of confidentiality. As you are also likely to be coding your data in the analysis stage it is very important that you know your coding system well, for example, disguised initials, as well as dating your transcripts, diary notes and tapes. If you do not establish good order now you run the very real risk later on of not being able to trace back who said what when.

At the end of the data collection phase of your study you will have a combination of some of the following: audiotape cassettes, videotape cassettes, interview transcripts, fieldnotes, supporting documentation (for example, minutes from meetings, job descriptions, policies and procedures), reflective accounts and possibly free text from questionnaires. The most important point at this stage is to *keep a clean, unmarked copy of everything; NEVER scribble on or cut up your only transcript*. Make copies of all original documentation apart from tape recordings, and put the originals in a safe place, clearly marked so that they cannot be mistaken for copies. It is advisable to make multiple copies of interview transcripts, the reason for which will become clear later. This is the stage when you will need to take over a large space or room, in which you can be confident that nobody will touch your work. Then you can arrange your data in a way that suits you, knowing you can at any time put your hand on the document you wish to retrieve.

Immersing yourself in the data

At this stage it is a good idea to simply immerse yourself in the data, reading and re-reading the transcripts and listening to your tape recordings over and over again. This is a fundamental stage in qualitative analysis. The only way to extract the true meaning of the data is to get as close to them as possible. However, there are several problems with this; in particular there is an assumption that you are doing the research full-time and therefore have the luxury of uninterrupted thought processes. In reality, many researchers are part time and find that no sooner have they begun to study the data than they have to return to the real world of the day job. Having said that, there is a problem with total immersion in 'not being able to see the wood for the trees'; you may find that you are so close to the data you can no longer hear what is being said. Riley (1990) talks about 'repetition and distancing' and suggests that every so often you come away from the data to reflect on it. In fact, it does not really matter that you are part-time (providing you have planned sufficient time for this stage and are not rushing your analysis) so long as you use the time you have constructively. Interview tapes can be listened to over and over again in the car, while cooking the dinner or in the bath. Bits of transcripts can be read on the bus or train or during a coffee or lunch break. Immersing yourself in the data while being a part-time researcher means keeping at it at every available opportunity. It also helps to talk out loud and to repeat phrases that seem significant.

Coding transcripts

Once engaged in this process you will want to begin to code your data. Essentially this means marking up your interview transcripts. There are a number of different ways of doing this but probably the easiest is to use different coloured highlighter pens. You need to code the person and the content. First, take a coloured pen and mark right down the margin of every page of the transcript, using a different colour for each person. This means that when you come to cut the pages up you can trace back who said what. Remember to keep a note of which colour margin is which interview.

Burnard (1991) then suggests that the transcripts are read through again and that as many headings as necessary are written down to describe all aspects of the content. This is known as 'open coding' and is the development of a category system which should account for almost all the data. You will then need to go through the transcripts yet again and in the opposite margin attribute categories to the text. At this stage it does not matter if you feel you have too many categories but it is important to categorise all the data. There will also be a 'dross' category; these are the conversational fillers, as well as 'umm, well, could you repeat the question please?' which can be discarded.

Hearing what the data has to say

This process of data analysis assumes that you are not using pure grounded theory but are using semi-structured interviews as one of your research methods. Unstructured data is quite different and the analysis takes place as you go along, relating the themes from one encounter to the next. This is known as 'theoretical sampling'. Such a process may result in some structured data capture in another phase of the study. However, even when conducting semi-structured interviews, making notes in the field and so on, you are bound to be doing some informal analysis as you go along. This is perfectly reasonable and indeed necessary, for until you recognise the same themes recurring again and again during your data collection phase you will be unsure that you have gathered enough. This is known as 'saturation' and is a perennial problem in qualitative research given the often small numbers in the sample group; how do you know when you have got enough data? Folklore has it that one famous social researcher pinned large envelopes on the wall around his study each labelled with a category which he would fill up as he gathered more and more data. The category reached saturation when the envelope fell off the wall!

So while some analysis is expected as you go along there is always the danger that you prejudice the data either because you had a hunch before you conducted the research and are just dying to expose it or because a theme seems to be emerging which really excites you even though you have not put it to the test. This is very difficult to deal with but you must try hard at this stage only to give categories headings and not jump several stages ahead trying to infer anything significant.

'Within the broad theme of lay participation in care I got very excited about what appeared to be the significance of the body and touching the body when washing or giving nursing care. Before I knew it I was discussing this category with my supervisor and a colleague who was expert in this field and really thought I was on to something. In the end it was a complete red herring which was only exposed when my final categories didn't fit the data. It was nothing to do with the body it was to do with who was giving what care. I could have saved myself a lot of time and anxiety if I hadn't tried to jump ahead of myself.'

Linda Crofts

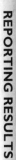

Collapsing the categories

Collapsing the categories is described by Burnard (1991) as the grouping together of categories under higher order headings. So, for example, you may have around twenty categories which might collapse down into four or five broader categories. There are several ways to do this but my own preferred method is to 'cut and paste'. This requires cutting up the coded transcripts and placing them in little piles on a large table under their category headings. You can

Raw data categories

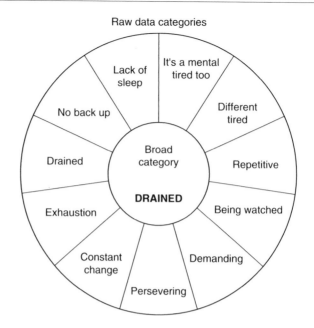

Fig. 10.3 *'Becoming a mother' (Barclay et al., 1997, from Blackwell publishers with permission)*

then manipulate the piles around the table until you begin to see some connections. Figure 10.3 shows an example from the study 'Becoming a mother'. In this study some sixty categories were collapsed into six. The example given is 'Drained'.

When the data do not fit

Although in theory the categories should collapse quite neatly, in practice you may find that you are left with stray piles around the table that do not seem to fit anywhere. This can be for a number of reasons; it may be that you have tried to prejudice the data and you need to go back to the drawing broad and regroup your categories, or indeed you may need to reinterpret the transcripts completely and start all over again (hence the need for multiple copies of transcripts). You may find that you do not have enough data and that you are nowhere near saturation. In this case you will need to collect more. However, if you have done everything right up to now it may just be that you are waiting for the breakthrough. If this is the case then go away and do something else, then maybe listen to the tapes again to remind yourself of the context and hope that inspiration will come.

'I was left with four categories that didn't seem to fit anywhere and were not saying what I expected them to say. There were a few quotes among them in particular that really bothered me so I went back and listened to the tape. There was something about the way the nurse said the same words over again. Lightning struck when I was hanging out the washing; it had taken so long because I was so sure the data would say something else.'

Linda Crofts

If you are stuck, try pasting the cut-out paragraphs onto a large piece of paper grouped in their categories; sometimes seeing all the pieces together can trigger something. You will probably need to do this once you have completed your analysis anyway, just to restore order to all the bits of paper.

During this phase you can get a sense of the weighting of categories but it is worth pointing out that the larger categories may not be the most significant; indeed they may be doing little more than stating the obvious. It is the smaller categories that may be the most significant and move your analysis on from being simply descriptive to interpretative. The trouble is, as Riley (1990) explains, you can fall in love with your data because you live and breathe it and having to move on to analysis can be difficult because it requires you to stand back and let go to an extent.

Although your categories have been broadly derived from interview transcripts, it is vital to support this material with your field-notes, diary entries and other supporting documentation. No doubt you are hoping these entries support your findings but there may be contradictions. This is why it is important to triangulate data; what participants say at interview may not be entirely reliable and if other data contradict this then you need to consider how to write this up. In any event, before making your final judgements you need to refer back to your original master transcripts to ensure that you have not interpreted and classified the data entirely out of context.

This process can of course be assisted by the use of computer packages. New packages come on to the market quite frequently but at the time of writing WINMAX is a qualitative package that can help derive themes and categories from raw data entries. Some researchers feel that using computer packages is just as time-consuming as analysing by hand, but it is much neater and negates the need for piles of paper around the room.

When going through your transcripts it is very tempting to look for 'quotability' in the text, in other words to choose the best quotes to illustrate the theme. Again, it is very easy to make the data fit the quote rather than the other way round if you do this; you are better advised to wait until you have done a cut-and-paste after category classification and then choose the most significant quote.

Validating your data may take a number of forms. The university may require you to authenticate your work and therefore your supervisor may need evidence of your coded transcripts, fieldnotes and actual tapes. Others merely require you to sign a declaration of authenticity. However, you may also wish to validate your data through an independent party who will confirm that they arrive at the same interpretation of categories as you have. This remains controversial in that since qualitative research is not seeking objectivity it is debatable whether one person's interpretation can be compared to another. This is not an issue that will be discussed here; suffice to say that if it is an academic requirement that an independent party is used then ensure you have arranged this in good time.

Writing up the results

The traditional research process demands that data collection is followed by data analysis, description of findings, discussion, implications for practice, summary and conclusions. Once past the data collection phase this structure does not really work for qualitative studies. Instead it is far more logical to present results as shown in Table 10.8.

If you are not carrying out research as part of an academic course then you may wish to present your results in this way. An excellent example is given in the study by Barclay *et al.* (1997). However, if you are on an academic course then you must follow university guidance, which may mean having to present each part of each category under the traditional headings.

REPORTING RESULTS

Table 10.8 *Presenting results in qualitative studies*

Category 1	Category 2	Category 3	Category 4
Analysis	Analysis	Analysis	Analysis
Description of findings	Description of findings	Description of findings	Description of findings
Discussion	Discussion	Discussion	Discussion
Implications for practice	Implications for practice	Implications for practice	Implications for practice

Implications for practice

If you have conducted a modest research study then your recommendations for practice should be modest too. It is not appropriate to make sweeping recommendations for nursing practice when you conducted your study with a sample group of five. What you can do is recommend a larger study and you can certainly highlight the significance of your findings. If you have married your findings with a return to the literature then you are able to state that your findings are consistent with those of others.

KEY POINTS

✔ Do not confuse qualitative and quantitative methods of analysis; they are trying to do quite different things.

✔ Keep your data under control and in order. Always keep an unmarked master copy of transcripts.

✔ Beware of prejudicing the data when you come to classify it.

✔ Moving from the descriptive to the analytical can be difficult when you are so close to the data.

✔ Analysis can be computer assisted.

✔ Ensure your recommendations are consistent with the findings.

REFERENCES

Barclay, L., Everitt, L., Rogan, F., Schmied, V. and Wyllie, A. (1997) Becoming a mother – an analysis of women's experience of early motherhood. *Journal of Advanced Nursing* **25**: 719–728.

Burnard, P. (1991) A method of analysing interview transcripts in qualitative research. *Nurse Education Today* **11**: 461–466.

Guba, E.G. and Lincoln, Y.S. (1989) *Fourth Generation Evaluation*. Newbury Park, CA: Sage.

Morse, J.M. (ed.) (1991) *Qualitative Nursing Research*. Newbury Park, CA: Sage.

Nolan, M. and Behi, R. (1995a) Reliability: consistency and accuracy in measurement. *British Journal of Nursing* **4**(8): 472–475.

Nolan, M. and Behi, R. (1995b) Alternative approaches to establishing reliability and validity. *British Journal of Nursing* **4**(10): 587–590.

Nolan, M. and Behi, R. (1995c) Triangulation: the best of both worlds? *British Journal of Nursing* **4**(14): 829–832.

Polit, D.F. and Hungler, B.P. (1997) *Essentials of Nursing Research: Methods, Appraisal and Utilization*, 4th edition. Philadelphia: Lippincott.

Riley, J. (1990) *Getting the Most from your Data – a Handbook of Practical Ideas on How to Analyse Qualitative Data*. Bristol: Technical Educational Services.

11

DISSEMINATING RESEARCH FINDINGS

Maggie Tarling

- Disseminating the results of your research
- Publishing in journals
- Making presentations

INTRODUCTION

If you are conducting your research as part of an academic course you will need to produce a dissertation or thesis. This chapter does not propose to deal with the issue of dissertation/thesis preparation. Universities have specific guidelines on the presentation of your research. It is imperative to keep to these guidelines and seek the advice of your supervisor (see Chapter 1). However, you should seriously consider the wider dissemination of your hard work. If nursing is to become an evidence-based practice, there needs to be 'evidence' available for nurses to evaluate. Hicks (1995) suggested that there is a short-fall in published nursing research. This shortfall is due to a lack of confidence rather than a failure of nurses to conduct research (Hicks, 1994). As a researcher you have a moral obligation to disseminate the results of your research as they may have an impact upon patient care.

The dissemination of research findings is a critical aspect of the research process. Dissemination does not merely mean the publication of your work in a journal but the wider dissemination of your results to various audiences, such as the LREC, funding bodies, to other professional colleagues at conferences and meetings, both at local and national or indeed international level. The reasons for this are many. Bodies such as the LREC, funding bodies or your local R&D department have a vested interest in knowing how resources have been utilised and will require a report. If you want to have an impact upon care the most immediate vehicle by which to achieve this is to present work at conferences or appropriate meetings, such as the Local Health Authority or Regional Health Authority meetings. These venues open your research to critical review from professionals who may have an influence upon policy and change. These meetings are very important to enable you to increase your influence upon practice. It is equally important not to forget the staff and patients who may have helped you conduct your research in the first place. This is often forgotten and many nurses in practice are fed up with researchers who just seem to 'smash and grab' data and are never heard from again. Local meetings are a useful tool in helping you to feedback your results in your own areas. These meetings are also useful for helping you to practise your presentations before you present at larger conferences or meetings.

There are other 'political' reasons why you should seriously consider publishing your results in a journal. Research plays a major role in academic funding. This presents a particular challenge to many departments of nursing in higher education, as they have not performed terribly well overall in the last two Higher Education Funding Council Research Assessment Exercises (RAE) (Cooke and Green, 2000). The RAE uses the publishing rates of academic departments as a measure of research activity, and will allocate funds to university departments accordingly. The reasons for this poor performance in the RAE are many. Research is a relatively new activity in nursing and it takes time to establish the research expertise required to do well. Many of the old colleges of nursing were integrated into what were polytechnics, which did not traditionally have a strong research foundation. Nursing departments that were incorporated into the older universities have fared better because of the research tradition in these institutions.

There is a real need to establish a nursing research base. Part of the RAE not only looks at what other research funding has been attracted into a department but will also look at the quality of the research produced. There is a lot of debate about how the quality of research is measured, but one of the measures the RAE uses is the publication rate. How many papers are published? It is not enough just to publish your research anywhere; the quality of the journal is also taken into account. Good-quality journals that have a peer review process are evaluated highly.

Resources are limited and the researcher's life can be quite difficult at the best of times. Publication of results gives kudos to the author and having your paper peer reviewed also adds a dimension of validity to your research. Therefore where you publish is an important consideration and peer-reviewed journals are preferable. Having a record of publications can increase the likelihood of gaining funding (see Chapter 7) for subsequent research. If you are based in an academic institution then publication becomes an even more important issue. However, this can leave you with a dilemma. The RAE exercise does have a limited view of dissemination. When you come to disseminate the results of your research you need to consider your audience. Unfortunately the peer-reviewed journals, though highly regarded in the RAE process, are not necessarily very widely read by the general nursing population. Although a journal such as the *Nursing Times* has a wide readership, it would not compare favourably with a more academic journal in the eyes of the RAE. However, *Nursing Times* does publish abstracts from *NTResearch*, which is peer reviewed. It is possible to gain both academic kudos and a wider audience using this means.

Publication in a journal is only one element of research dissemination. You will need skills in writing research reports for LRECs, funding bodies and journals. You will also need to be able to prepare abstracts for conferences and meetings and to develop skills in giving poster presentations and presenting yourself and your work at conferences and meetings. What follows is a novice's guide to disseminating your research.

DISSEMINATION

There are general issues that are applicable to all the different methods of dissemination. It does not matter if you are writing a report for the MRC, an abstract for a conference, putting an oral presentation together, there are several general questions you need to consider before you start.

✔ The audience

Who is your audience? What is your audience's agenda? What are they interested in? What level of expertise do they have? Answering these questions will help you to set the level of language you will use. Will make sure that you focus upon the audience's needs and requirements.

✔ The purpose

What is your purpose? Do you have a particular message to get across? Answering these will help you to focus your message.

✔ Guidelines

Are there guidelines available to help you? If guidelines are available, you MUST follow them.

✔ *Resources*

Can you get hold of an example? Can you talk to someone with experience? Can you attend a meeting or conference before you present? These are all extremely useful experiences to tap into and can be extremely helpful.

THE RESEARCH REPORT

A research report is a summary of your research. It will generally contain an introduction, aims, literature review, design, methodology, ethical considerations, data analysis, conclusion and discussion. Most research reports will have this sort of structure. However, the length, the focus and other information may be different depending upon the audience the report is written for. For example, most if not all funding bodies require a research report to be written at the end of the funding agreement, for longer term projects there may be a requirement to produce several reports at different time scales during the research project. As well as the usual information required they will be particularly interested in how funds have been used and also how the research has been disseminated. They will be interested in any publications or presentations. They will also be interested in whether the original objectives of the research have been met and any actual or potential benefits your research may have. The MRC's web site gives useful information about the information they require for research reports (http://www.mrc.ac.uk).

The LREC or R&D department in your Trust equally require reports and it is important that you do not forget them. LRECs are also interested in whether you have met your objectives, what impact your research has or may have, whether you have used resources effectively and how you have disseminated your results. Each body will have their own guidelines on the structure of the research report and it is important to follow these. Not to do so may jeopardise any chances of further funding in the future.

PUBLICATION

First things first

✔ *Choosing the journal*

You will need to consider the relevant audience. Do you want to speak to nurses locally? Is there an in-house journal in your area?

Do you want to reach nurses in a specialist field or a wider audience?

✔ *Allowing time*

Be aware that the process of writing for publication is a long one. It *always* takes longer than you think.

Find out the gap between submission and publication, as this can be quite long. It can be more than a year in some cases.

✔ *Planning*

Each publication will have its own guidelines for authors submitting work. Do not assume that all journals have the same requirements. Failure to adhere to these may mean your paper gets returned to you unread. Each journal publishes its guidelines in issues of the journal, although not necessarily in each edition. Phone up and ask for these to be sent to you if you cannot locate them. Campbell (1998) has produced a useful guide for publishing in the *Journal of Advanced Nursing*.

If you are not sure that the journal you are considering will be interested in your work then it is wise to contact the editor to see if there will be an interest. This can sometimes save a lot of time.

Make sure that you have access to a decent computer. Journals will not accept handwritten scripts. Some journals will require the manuscript on disk as well. Make sure that the software you are using is compatible, including the version you are using.

If you are not good at proof-reading, get someone who is to check your work.

Preparing your manuscript

When you are writing the text of your research you should consider the points from Chapter 4 on reviewing the literature. Always keep in mind that others will use these sorts of assessments when reviewing your work.

It is imperative to comply with the journal's guidelines, e.g. size of margin, double spacing, style of referencing. Otherwise you may find that your manuscript is returned unread.

It is worth taking great care with the title and the abstract. These are the two mechanisms by which your paper will be accessed by others (see Chapter 3). The title should reflect the problem/hypothesis you

> **Box 11.1** *Citing from the World Wide Web*
>
> **Citing a website:**
>
> The MRC has a useful website on applying for funding (http://www.mrc.ac.uk)
>
> **Citing specific documents:**
>
> 'For example the NHS Centre for Reviews and Dissemination (2001) gives guidance on reviewing qualitative research.'
>
> **This would be cited in the reference list as:**
>
> NHS Centre for Reviews and Dissemination (2001) Undertaking Systematic Reviews of Research on Effectiveness: CRD's Guidance for Carrying Out or Commissioning Reviews (CRD Report 4: 2nd Edition). York: NHS Centre for Reviews and Dissemination. Available from: http://www.york.ac.uk/inst/crd/report4.htm

looked at, the methodology you used and the subjects you investigated. The abstract should summarise your aims, your methods, your subjects and the results. Many journals will also ask for up to six keywords associated with your research to aid in library indexing.

It is also important to be careful with references and follow the guidelines from the particular journal you are submitting to. With the increasing accessibility of the World Wide Web the amount of information available is expanding at a rapid rate. You may find that you want to cite from Web sources. However, you must always be careful when using information from the Web, as there is little or no control as to what information is published. You must be sure about the credibility of the author and the source of information.

You may want to cite a whole website or specific documents or part of a web document. Box 11.1 gives some idea of how to cite this sort of information. The American Psychological Association (2000) has some useful guidance on citing from the World Wide Web. However, as always, you should check with the appropriate journal about their own policy.

What happens to your manuscript?

A manuscript submitted to a journal will usually go through the following stages prior to publication:

- Your manuscript will be received by the editor. An assessment will be made as to whether the research will fit with the interest of the journal. If it does not or the manuscript is obviously inadequately prepared then it will be returned to you.

- If the manuscript follows the guidelines and the editor considers the research to be of interest then the manuscript is sent for review. The autobiographical data is removed and the body of the manuscript is sent off to the relevant reviewers. Journals who use the review process will have a list of individuals with expertise in different areas who act as reviewers for the journal. The process is anonymous. Neither you nor the reviewers will know each other.
- The editor will make a decision about your paper in light of the reviewers' comments. The editor has the final decision, which will be either to accept, accept with amendments (most common) or reject.
- Usually the manuscript is returned to you with the reviewers' comments and the decision of the editor. If accepted, you most probably will have to make amendments to the paper.
- If your paper is rejected outright
  - Then there may have been a fundamental flaw in your research and there is nothing much you can do about it at this stage.
  - Or your research did not fit the interests of the journal. Therefore consider submitting to another one.
- Once you have returned the paper to the editor, it goes into production and you will receive a proof copy to read before publication.
- You should also receive a limited number of offprints once the paper is published.

This process varies between journals, especially where the journal does not use the reviewing process. However, you can appreciate that this process may take some time before you see your name in print.

PRESENTING AT MEETINGS

'It takes courage to stand up and speak and another sort to sit and listen. If research means anything to you, you will learn to do both and accept the consequences.' (Calnan, 1976)

It does take courage to present your findings to others. You have often spent a long time planning and conducting your research and it almost becomes 'your baby'. It then becomes difficult to allow others to criticise what you have done. It can almost feel personal. But the value of research only comes into focus when others have a chance to hear and evaluate your results. In order to survive the analysis of your work, you should take the view that any criticism is not personal, and foster a confidence and belief in your work. One of the most immediate ways of presenting your results is at a conference or meeting. These venues can range from small seminar groups within your local area to large conferences. There is great value in attending and presenting research at meetings as you can encounter others doing the same sort of research and reap the benefits of networking with like-minded people. There are several factors to consider before you submit your work for presentation.

- ✔ Who will benefit most from your results?
- ✔ Is there a relevant interest/professional group conference held?
- ✔ When are meetings held?
- ✔ Where are meetings held?
- ✔ Who will pay for travelling/accommodation costs?
- ✔ When is the deadline for submissions?
- ✔ Are there guidelines available about how to submit?
- ✔ Apply for the appropriate forms.

It is important to consider these questions before you start. If at all possible, it is worth attending a meeting before you have to present so that you can get an idea about what sort of research is presented, what other people do and the type of questions people ask.

There are two ways of presenting work at meetings, a verbal presentation or a poster presentation. The poster presentation is generally a more gentle way into presentation for the beginner, as you do not have to speak in front of a large number of people, which can be daunting to the uninitiated. There are simple steps that can be taken which make the process easier. Both types of presentation share common principles in preparation. What follows is a step-by-step guide to planning and giving a presentation at a meeting.

Planning

There are a few simple questions you need to ask before you actually start writing your poster or talk. First, it is important to consider your aims carefully in presenting your results. For example, do you want as many people as possible to know about your results? Is there a specific specialist group of individuals who would most benefit from your results? Such questions will identify your audience. This will in turn help you decide which meeting to submit your work to. You will see calls for papers advertised in the nursing press at various intervals.

DISSEMINATING RESEARCH FINDINGS

Box 11.2 *Abstract format*

Title	Keep short and descriptive of what you have done.
Introduction	Keep simple. State the problem and why you investigated it.
Methods	Describe what you did.
Results	Keep to the most relevant results. If you can use a table or chart do so.
Conclusion	State a short summary of your conclusions and possible areas for further research.
References	Quote a small number of most relevant references. The number allowed will vary.

The abstract

Many research meetings will require the submission of an abstract of your work. Some but not all meetings use the abstract as a basis for a peer review before it is accepted. Some meetings will publish the abstracts of meetings as a record.

The abstract is usually of limited length. This will vary between different meetings, from 200 to 400 words. They will issue a guideline as to how they want the abstract written. Be careful as different meetings have different requirements. So do not assume that all abstracts are done the same way. Most follow the format shown in Box 11.2.

The abstract you write will be the basic foundation for your poster or verbal presentation. Your presentation will allow you to expand on several points.

The presentation

Consider the following questions:

✔ *Who* will be in the audience. This knowledge will enable you to gauge the level of your presentation. If you are presenting to a specialist audience it will not be necessary to spend time explaining concepts and methods you may have used. However, if your audience does not have a background in your area of research then you will need to spend time defining what you did in more detail.

Where will the talk be given? The venue is important and will indicate the style of presentation. Presenting to a large audience is very different to presenting to a small informal group. You will also have to establish what audio-visual aids will be available to you. Never assume that a venue will have the equipment you require or that it will be in working order on the day.

 How much time do you have? Time is usually a limiting factor. You may only have ten minutes or you may have an hour. Obviously you need to consider which points to emphasize when time is very limited.

Answering the *who, where* and *time* questions informs the *what* question. The *what* refers to what you are going to talk about.

Structuring your presentation

Needless to say, a presentation, whether it is a poster or a verbal presentation, should have a beginning, a middle and an end. You should clearly state the problem, research question or hypothesis at the beginning. Then state what you looked at and how. State the results you found and finally discuss the implications of your results. This basic structure should allow for most research designs, whether qualitative or quantitative.

The poster presentation

The basic headings that you used for your abstract can be used as a guide to making the poster. However, the poster gives an opportunity to expand on the detail of the abstract. There is no right or wrong way of putting a poster presentation together but here are a few guidelines.

 Never underestimate the time it will take to make the poster. It *always* takes longer than you think it will. So do not leave it until the evening before to put it together.

 Make things simple.

Use pictures to display results, whenever possible. So use pie charts, graphs, photographs, illustrations whenever you can.

Use colour or bold print to highlight important points.

It is best to design your poster on a PC. This makes it easy to divide the poster into A4 size sections.

If it is possible to get your pages laminated do so. It becomes easier to transport the poster and set it up at the venue.

 It may be of use to produce a handout of your poster to give to delegates for further information. Or you may want to have a book available for people's comments.

Check what facilities will be available to you when you get there. How are posters set up? Will you need to bring pins or adhesives with you? You do not want to get to a venue and find that you cannot attach your poster.

 Remember you will need to be available by the poster to answer questions and discuss your research during the meeting.

The verbal presentation

This can be a more daunting experience but well worth the effort and preparation. When giving a verbal presentation it is far better to talk directly to the audience without the distraction of reading from a script. It looks more natural if you are speaking to the audience and are able to maintain eye contact. In order to do this well you will need to practise, practise, practise to give a polished performance. It is also a very good idea to use audio–visual aids (AVAs) as they give the audience something to look at, and are very useful in illustrating concepts and acting as an aide-mémoire for your talk. When planning your talk it is useful to structure your talk in a logical order (Figure 11.1).

Choosing an audio-visual aid

There are several options open to you. However, there is one that you are stuck with, that is, yourself. You are the first AVA the audience will see and notice. It is therefore important to consider the presentation of yourself. You should consider how you will dress for the occasion, how you will project yourself, as your credibility will to some extent be judged by how you present yourself. You will need to practise your talk beforehand and this is a good opportunity for others to let you know if you have any funny 'nervous twitches'. We all have nervous habits, such as, pacing, fiddling with pointers, pens, stuttering, going 'ummm' during pauses in speech. These nervous habits can actually make you more nervous and can be very distracting to an audience. (I once counted the number of times a lecturer of mine took off his glasses during a one-hour lecture. It was 21 times. Needless to say I can't remember the lecture but the glasses are a

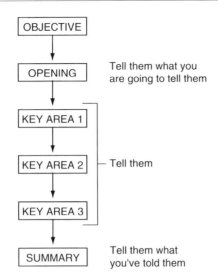

Fig. 11.1 *Structuring your presentation*

Box 11.3 *Audio-visual aids*	
White boards	Are useful for small group/seminar work. Need a marker and eraser.
Flip charts	Are useful for small group/seminar work. Need a marker but have the advantage of being quick; no need to erase work.
Overhead projector (OHP)	Can prepare work beforehand. Useful for larger audiences.
Slides	Can be prepared beforehand and can give a professional finish.
Video	Can be used to dramatic effect to illustrate a point.
Multimedia	Can produce a combination of all of the above using various software packages, such as PowerPoint.

vivid memory!) It is very difficult to eradicate these habits. It takes a lot of time and practice to polish presentation skills. However, you need to be aware of them before you can do anything about them.

The choice of AVA (Box 11.3) depends upon the venue you are going to present at and the type of presentation you will make.

If you are presenting to a small group or at a seminar and the style of presentation will involve the audience then white boards and flip charts are useful tools. They can be used to build on concepts and ideas as the presentation progresses. The main disadvantage is that there is only a limited amount of preparation that can be done beforehand. If your presentation is to a much larger audience, where there will be a limited amount of interaction during the presentation, then the other AVAs mentioned above will suit your purpose. Their main advantage is that they can all be prepared beforehand and can easily be transported to the venue. They can also give a professional look to a presentation. There are many computer packages available to produce OHPs, slides and multimedia presentations and they are well worth getting access to if at all possible.

Designing slides and OHPs

If you have not done this before it is best to get advice from someone who has had experience of producing these. If you do not have access to slide-making equipment it may be possible to get help from departments such as medical illustration or an AVA department

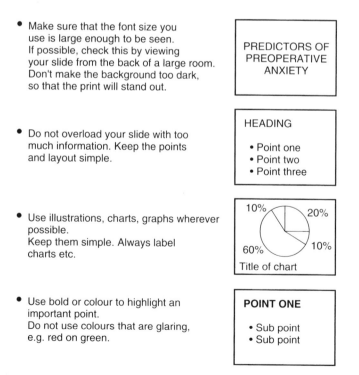

Fig. 11.2 *Designing slides*

which might be available in your hospital. Figure 11.2 gives a few guidelines to help in designing your slides/OHPs.

Designing a multimedia presentation

The general rules above also apply to this type of presentation. However, you do have a wider scope with a package such as PowerPoint as it enables you to use different sorts of effects. You can hide bullet points until you are ready to talk about them. You can use different effects to expose text when you want to. You can use video clips, sound effects and clip art that can move. There are all sorts of effects that can be used with this approach that can make your presentation interesting and have an impact.

Though the use of multimedia is now much more common and is very convenient (all you need to transport is a disk), you need to use it with caution. If you have not got a lot of experience the best advice is to keep it simple. Do not go for complicated special effects that could go wrong. If you do get an expert to design the presentation make sure that you have had a lot of practice using it so that you are very familiar with how it works and what to do if it goes wrong. I have seen many a speaker panic when the wrong key has been pressed and the screen disappears.

Always have a back-up presentation, such as OHPs, as computers have been known to crash. You may get to the venue and find that the software version you have used is not compatible. You must always check what versions of software the computer will run. It is also important to check that alternative AVAs are actually available.

Tips for using audio-visual aids

 Always make sure that you know how to work the AVA. Do you know how to turn on the OHP, slide projector, video, computer?

 Is there a suitable power source (relevant for smaller venues)?

Are the extras available, e.g. a marker pen for flip charts/marker boards, a pointer for OHPs and slides?

Does the equipment actually work?

Are your slides put in the right way up?

 Try not to be too clever. The more equipment you use the greater the probability that it will go wrong in the middle of your talk.

Check all equipment before your presentation. Get to the venue early so that you can use the AVA to make sure that it works; that your OHPs/slides will appear in the right order, that you have pointers, etc. If things are not working you will then have time to sort them out.

 Make sure there is an alternative AVA you could use if all goes wrong.

✔ Make sure you position yourself so that you will not obstruct the information presented.

 'Don't assume that equipment will be working on the day. At one venue the slide projector wasn't working. I had to muddle through with out-of-focus slides. Needless to say the talk wasn't a success.'

'I had done all my preparation and was feeling quite confident. However, I had assumed that as there was a slide projector that there would also be a pointer. I was wrong. It is very difficult to point to items on a projected slide. In the end I was lucky as someone else lent me their pointer.'

Maggie Tarling

Tackling nerves

No matter how many times you present at meetings you will experience nerves. Even the most seasoned presenters will confess, when pushed, that they experience anxiety before a presentation. A certain level of anxiety is a good motivator. However, you do not want your nervousness to interfere with your presentation.

Anxiety can affect people's performance in many ways. Commonly it affects the voice and can make your hands shake. This is unfortunate when you are going to give a talk. The best way of controlling these symptoms and giving a polished performance is to use little confidence tricks. Consider how you stand. Make sure that you stand upright as this will improve the projection of your voice. Slowing down your breathing will help to reduce the nervousness in your voice. Taking a slow deep breath before you start will help to centre you and calm you down. If your hands do shake make sure that you do not hold any pieces of paper as this will accentuate the problem. It is useful if you can stand behind a podium as you can rest your hands there and this will help you resist any nervous habits you may have. The podium is also a useful psychological barrier between yourself and the audience, you will not feel so exposed. If there is no podium it is important that you resist any urges to pace up and down or move about too much, as these nervous habits can be very distracting for the audience. Lastly, it is important to practise so that you are confident about the content of your presentation and about using the AVAs you have chosen. You will therefore have less to worry about. If something does go wrong do not panic; slow down or stop until the problem is sorted out.

Using humour

Using humour in a presentation can be extremely effective in getting the audience on your side and making your presentation memorable. However, this approach can be potentially disastrous. I would suggest only using humour if you feel very confident about your subject and your presentation skills. Only use this approach if you are familiar with the audience. You do not need to know the audience personally but you need an understanding of 'where they are coming from'.

Humour can be used in several different ways. From using a cartoon or humorous slide, making comments around the topic, but never, ever tell a joke unless you are good at them. Humour can be useful where you feel that the audience may potentially be antagonistic to your material and it is useful in 'breaking the ice' and building a bridge between yourself and the audience. Humour can also be effective in averting total disaster if you have any major technical hitches. Humour is a very powerful tool but must be used with caution as it can go disastrously wrong and there is nothing worse than standing on stage facing stony silence when you have just made what you think is the wittiest comment anyone has ever made.

Taking questions

At the end of your presentation there will be a period for taking questions from the audience. This can be quite daunting, as you have no control over this stage of events. You need to be aware that there are several different types of questioner. There are those who are genuinely interested in your research and will ask relevant questions. Then there are those who have their own agenda who want to make a general point within the forum you are presenting at. They usually start with 'I/We found that ...'. Whatever question you are asked, take a deep breath and consider the question carefully. If the question is unclear ask for it to be repeated. If you do not know the answer say so. This is where having a colleague in the audience can be useful.

KEY POINTS

Publication

 Choose the right journal for your audience.

 Contact the editor if you are unsure whether the journal will be interested in your work.

 Allow plenty of time for writing. It *always* takes longer than you think.

 Obtain the relevant guidelines for authors.

 Consider the guidelines for critiquing research (see Chapter 4) when writing your own paper.

 Write the title and abstract for your paper very carefully (see Chapter 3).

Presenting

 Try and attend a meeting before presenting.

 Practise, practise, practise beforehand. Practise at work, at home, in front of colleagues, the family, the cat, anyone who will listen. Practise until you are bored with it.

 Only use AVAs you are familiar with.

Keep things simple.

Get there early to ensure that equipment is available and working.

Take a deep breath before you start.

Do not rush yourself.

 Do not panic if something goes wrong. Stop and see if it can be sorted out. If not, carry on as best you can. A sense of humour is critical at this stage.

Have a colleague in the audience. It is good moral support.

Try and relax. It is possible to enjoy presenting your work.

REFERENCES

American Psychological Association (2000) Electronic reference formats recommended by the American Psychological Association. Available from: http://www.apa.org/journals/webref.html

Calnan, J. (1976) *One Way To Do Research: The A–Z For Those Who Must*. London: William Heinemann.

Campbell, G.C. (1998) Helping you get published in the Journal of Advanced Nursing. *Journal of Advanced Nursing* **28**(1): 8–9.

Cooke, A. and Green, B. (2000) Developing the research capacity of departments of nursing and midwifery based in higher education: a review of the literature. *Journal of Advanced Nursing* **32**(1): 57–65.

Hicks, C. (1994) Of sex and status: a study of the effects of gender and occupation on nurses' evaluations of nursing research. *Journal of Advanced Nursing* **17**: 1343–1349.

Hicks, C. (1995) The shortfall in published research: A study of nurses' research and publication activities. *Journal of Advanced Nursing* **21**: 594–604.

12

CAREERS IN RESEARCH

Joyce E. Kenkre

- Background
- Choice of career direction
- Applications and interviews

INTRODUCTION

Research conducted by nurses is not a new initiative. In 1857 Florence Nightingale prepared a report for the Royal Sanitary Commission, which included a thousand pages of printed tables and statistics (Baly, 1980). She compared the mortality and morbidity rates of men in the army to those in the surrounding area, and found that the mortality rate was twice as high in the army barracks, despite the fact that these were supposed to be fit men. Consequently, Florence Nightingale is considered not only an inspirational person by nurses but by statisticians too. The information gained from her research enabled her to prepare a factual report to present to the Commission.

Unfortunately, nurses as a professional body did not capitalise on this precedent but continued to be trained in a traditional manner. It was not until 1932 that post-registration Diplomas in Nursing were available in London and Leeds (Weir, 1996) and a further 30 years before the first degree course for nurses in the UK commenced in 1960, at the University of Edinburgh, 115 years after Florence Nightingale had presented her research-based report. The Briggs Report (Committee on Nursing, 1972) highlighted the need to bring 'research mindedness' into the curriculum and suggested that nursing should become a research-based profession. It is not before time that we as a profession base our practice on research-based evidence.

It is acknowledged that nursing is considered to be a newcomer in the research arena by comparison with other clinical specialties. One explanation could be that nursing, as a largely female group, sometimes experiences an 'invisibility' syndrome in male-dominated institutions such as higher education. Nursing can become absorbed into existing university structures and is sometimes not accepted as a discrete discipline in its own right. This can result in a limitation of access to research funding, career and promotion blockages and a failure to recognise the importance of the research and development agenda for nurses. However, it is important for us as a professional body to develop our research expertise, so that we become acknowledged researchers in our own right and selected as collaborators of choice by our colleagues. Therefore, it is essential to identify the role of research within existing career pathways as well as creating new innovative ways of negotiating the research journey in order for nurses and nursing to be able to fulfil their true potential.

ACADEMIC CAREER

Nurses who decide that they would like to develop an academic career may do so to teach or to develop a research career. If a nurse predominantly wishes to teach in higher education, this would normally entail completing a teaching qualification prior to applying for a lecturing post. However, this is not a mandatory requirement to teach in higher education. It is expected that a person in a lecturing position should be able to critically appraise research papers and be able to teach students in the light of research evidence. Nurse lecturers are increasingly being actively encouraged to conduct research. Indeed, to be able to progress up this career pathway at the highest level research grants and publications are a necessary requirement.

Conversely, a nurse wishing to particularly develop a career in research would apply for research positions within university departments. Starting as a research assistant/associate, the nurse will be involved in a range of activities in the practical conduct of research such as the organisation, data collection, data management including coding, the input of data and preliminary analysis and assisting with writing of reports.

The normal progression along this career pathway is to lecturer grade or research fellow. The research activities at this level would involve some of the practical management of research projects, the writing of protocols with a senior academic, preparation of reports and publications for journals and the dissemination of information at conferences. At the next level a senior lecturer/fellow should be an acknowledged researcher at a national level and have publications in international journals. The researcher in this position would be developing new research projects, leading grant applications, publishing high-quality research and guiding junior members of research staff.

The position of reader is bestowed on an individual who has gained an international reputation for research in a particular area and this post enables the holder to develop their area of knowledge and expertise further. The lead for research within an academic department is usually held by a professor.

Nurses are now being recognised for their strategic organisational skills and are now gaining positions as Deans (administrative heads) of Schools or of administrative areas within universities such as research. Today there are great opportunities for nurses to develop their career within the academic setting.

CLINICAL RESEARCH NURSE CAREER

Many nurses start their career in research as a clinical research nurse (CRN), and the development of skills and knowledge required to conduct numerous multi-centre clinical therapeutic trails provides an excellent grounding in the discipline, organisation and management of research conducted to recognised international standards. A clinical therapeutic trial is the prospective study of medicinal products in human subjects. These are normally categorised into four phases, the first of which is the initial introduction of the drug into human subjects to monitor any effect the drug may have on the body. The second phase is a series of randomised placebo-controlled trials to determine if the new product has any therapeutic effect on patients with a specified condition. The third phase of studies used to determine the dose range and therapeutic effect of the drug compared with other established treatments for the conditions being treated. The fourth phase consists of formal post-marketing surveillance studies conducted to monitor for toxicity of the new compound in a larger number of patients.

Nurses in the clinical setting undertaking research activities should be graded appropriately, taking into account the additional knowledge, skills and responsibility associated with their role in research. Hence, a junior 'D' grade nurse who is given research responsibilities should be paid as an 'E' grade. A nurse starting into the clinical research role would be expected to work under close supervision, identify and screen suitable patients for the trials in progress, carry out procedures, take patient samples, undertake treatment interventions according to a predetermined protocol. On the management of the research information the nurse needs to ensure that the collection of data meets the desired standard, that the data, if required, are entered onto a computer ensuring patient confidentiality. It is important that the informed consent process is ongoing throughout a trial or study, as the physical and mental needs of the patient are paramount.

As the CRN gains more knowledge, skills and experience they will be expected to work with a degree of autonomy, frequently conducting concurrent research studies. The CRN would be expected to liaise with the sponsoring companies, other departments involved in the research such as pharmacy, laboratory staff, and technicians as well as the immediate multi-disciplinary research teams within the department. The CRN has an active role in ethical requirements including ethics committee submissions, the informed consent process and patient support. As the nurse at this level is not working in an assistant capacity this should be reflected in the clinical grading ('F' grade).

The next grade for the CRN would be considered as a clinical specialist within their field of practice ('G' grade). The nurse would have a research, educational and developmental role within the research projects. The nurse at this stage should be considering undertaking post-registration education in clinical research at certificate level with progression to masters level.

A CRN at 'H' grade must have the ability to lead in the development, assessment and supervision of research protocols. The organisation and management of resources, financial negotiation for the cost of protocols, negotiation of contracts for members of the research team are important elements of the position. As the nursing lead and a specialist in the field of practice the CRN at this level would be accountable for the nursing elements within the research being conducted, the application of research and the dissemination and publication of research findings.

Many research units are now managed and/or led by nurses ('I' grade). These nurses have key responsibilities, which include responsibility for large multi-disciplinary teams of health care professionals in the conduct of international trials, building capacity and infrastructure to be able to conduct quality research, actively developing and promoting the institutional research agenda and leading by example in terms of research activity and publications. These nurses have a wealth of experience, although a higher degree is also desirable, either in research methods and/or business administration.

CLINICAL CAREER

Although the clinical grading within primary care and secondary care trusts at present is based on variations of the Whitley NHS

Clinical Grading Scales, this no longer demonstrates the changing roles of nurses within their clinical careers. This clinical career pathway is considered an exciting development for nurses who wish to expand clinical expertise and practice to consultant nurse level. The development of evidence-based practice requires highly skilled and competent researchers, and highly skilled and competent individuals are unlikely to be attracted to research if there is no clear and agreed career and pay structure.

Newly qualified nurses will initially be consolidating their knowledge, skills and expertise within their field of practice. Basing their clinical practice on research evidence with a questioning approach, which may raise research questions, should be an important component of this consolidation process. Nurses should be reading and appraising research-based literature, have opportunities for continuing education and participation in specialist interest groups. Nurses within their clinical practice should have the facility to be involved in some element of the research process to aid in their development.

Nurses working at this higher level, as nurse practitioners or clinical nurse specialists should be facilitating evidence-based practice founded on relevant quality research. Nurses at this level may be working in specific clinical areas such as primary care, A&E, occupational health, walk-in centres or with particular patient groups such as the homeless, breast care, ENT or drug dependency. The advanced practitioner assumes clinical responsibility for his or her own patients/clients caseload. The nurse will typically screen for early signs of disease and risk factors, diagnose undifferentiated conditions, and devise integrated care plans, which includes nursing and medical management of care. It is important that as practitioners, nurses identify gaps in their knowledge and expertise, so they can be addressed.

Responsible for incorporating high-quality research evidence into patient care, it is acknowledged that consultant nurses are to be the future clinical leaders within their field of expertise. These nurses have to combine the clinical role with a strategic and operational one. The role has four core functions (Department of Health, 1999): expert practice; professional leadership and consultancy; education, training and development; and practice and service development, research and evaluation. These new consultant posts are frequently in conjunction with academic institutions so that a nurse with advanced clinical expertise will have the opportunity to develop personally with the prospect of being able to undertake a clinical doctorate. This academic qualification will give the consultant nurse the expertise to conduct or assimilate research to base their practice on evidence.

RESEARCH SUPPORT/MANAGEMENT CAREER

Commissioning and funding bodies employ people to administer their research funding programmes. This is a career where nurses can use their clinical and/or research expertise and knowledge in the development and support of research undertaken in academic and clinical settings. Nurses in these positions play an important role in assisting other nurses to develop their research capacity and capability to enable them to deliver relevant quality research to base their practice. The NHS R&D programme has facilitated the development of research support and management roles through funding of geographically based academic R&D support units to provide support and guidance to less experienced researchers. These nurses often have broad research experience and use their knowledge and skills to help others. At the same time, Research Management Offices have been established in many NHS Trusts to oversee the use of funds from the R&D Levy, and nurses often fill these administrative posts.

The research assistant/associate or research nurse is the beginning position on this career pathway in the support and administration of programmatic research activity. In this role they may write briefing papers on particular topics to support decision making or as a research provider may support and co-ordinate research activity by others, or may be involved in supporting the 'D' for development and the utilisation of research findings.

The next steps along this career pathway are as either research officer/fellow or senior research officer/fellow over time. These research support staff will probably take the position of project lead in support and administration of programmatic research activity; and will also be expected to contribute to strategic development.

At the executive level the principal research officer or research director is expected to provide strong scientific input into operational activities, have overall responsibility and a broad overview of organisational and management activity, and provide strong strategic lead to the organisation. This research support/management pathway is, for example, to develop the infrastructure within an NHS Trust or to work directly for research sponsors in a scientific support role.

PHARMACEUTICAL INDUSTRY CAREER

Experienced clinical research nurses (CRNs) frequently seek employment within the pharmaceutical industry due to career prospects and financial reward. Following a period of training the clinical research associate is assigned to specific investigator sites to organise the requirements of the study site staff to enable them to conduct a clinical trial to an acceptable standard. These investigator sites may be anywhere in the world, so the clinical research associate has to be prepared to undertake a great deal of air travel. Both the pharmaceutical industry staff and the site personnel work to predefined standard operating procedures for their company or institution to ensure the research is conducted to international standards of good clinical practice.

The more senior clinical research associates have the added responsibility of leading teams monitoring programmes of research. As with any field team structure, communication and dissemination of information is an important part of their role. Another of their responsibilities is the development of research protocols and study specific documentation, which can be used internationally. Project managers will have responsibility for the resourcing of research programmes at an international level.

OTHER RESEARCH CAREERS

Other related careers where nurses may utilise their research expertise include medical writer and auditor. These are usually very well paid and many people undertaking these roles choose to work in a freelance capacity.

Medical writer

One of the benefits of this career is the ability to work from home, although very short time scales make this a highly pressured job. Medical writing can involve writing up specific research reports, manuscripts, patient information leaflets or other documentation required by pharmaceutical or related companies.

Auditor

The role of the auditor is to check that a clinical therapeutic trial has been conducted to the standard required by good clinical practice and that all the documentation from the initial visit to completion is above reproach. The auditor may be employed by the pharmaceutical company or by a regulatory agency.

DEVELOPMENT OF QUALIFICATIONS

It is important when considering your future career to ascertain which qualifications (clinical, research or business) would be most beneficial to you, or indeed whether you can obtain a qualification that will encompass all of these. There are now numerous master degree programmes available within specialist areas, all of which will have a research element. More nurses are looking to undertake post-graduate education at doctorate level, which can include a doctorate by portfolio or a clinical taught doctorate.

JOB APPLICATIONS

Advertisements for jobs within the different career pathways can be found in a variety of newspapers, journals and websites (Box 12.1). These are scrutinised by individuals interested in applying for certain posts but also by others wishing to gain information about staff movement in other departments, funding gained for projects or knowledge about areas that other departments potentially wish to develop.

The advertisement will usually give you an outline of the job, where to apply to for an application form and a contact person for informal discussion. If you are seriously considering applying, it is advisable to make an appointment for an informal discussion. This meeting should give you sufficient knowledge about the post, the other staff that you would be working with and the potential for

---

Box 12.1 *Sources of job advertisements*

- RCN R&D Co-ordinating Centre http://www.man.ac.uk/rcn/
- *Nursing Standard*
- *RCN Bulletin*
- *Guardian* (Tuesday and Wednesday)
- *Nursing Times*
- *Health Services Journal*
- *CRF Clinical Research Focus*
- *Daily Telegraph* (Thursday)
- *New Scientist*

CAREERS IN RESEARCH

development within the position. During these discussions you should have been given some indication whether you would be suitable to apply for the position, and equally have decided whether you would want to apply for the post.

Job applications usually list skills and knowledge that are essential and those that are desirable. If an applicant meets all of the essential requirements and some of the desirable ones then they should be considered for interview. It is wise when applying for a position to read through the instructions and requirements for any job carefully and comply with them as in the most competitive positions any simple breach may lead to exclusion.

CURRICULUM VITAE (CV)

On completion of the job application form, there is frequently a request for supporting information, often in the form of a curriculum vitae (CV). A CV is simply a document that illustrates your achievements and abilities, in order to demonstrate your suitability for the job advertised. Employers have normally specified the essential and desirable characteristics required for the job, so in reading your CV they need to know that you meet these necessary requirements.

Nurses that have been involved in academic life for the majority of their career may have long and detailed master CVs. However, if you submit a very long, detailed CV it may be that the selection panel will miss the major points due to the inclusion of too much minor detail. In this case it may be better to consider being selective in the content. An applicant may consider placing a one page résumé at the front of their CV citing, for example, five key achievements, five key abilities and qualifications. However, there are some necessary components which would include: educational background, qualifications, previous appointments, teaching experience, research experience, research grant income, publications, conference presentations, guest lectures/plenary presentations, chair and membership of committees (regionally, national and international), membership of organisations and educational courses taken. It would not be expected for junior academic staff to have experience in all these areas but this may give them an insight into areas needed to be developed to advance their career.

Applicants usually have to supply the names of referees. Your present employer is usually considered mandatory for inclusion, however, you should consider strategically the choice of other referees in support of your application.

INTERVIEW

Any information stated within your application is open for questioning during the interview process, so do not be tempted to include anything that cannot be substantiated! It is often said that the decision on who gets a job is actually decided within the first 30 seconds of an interview, so wear something that you feel comfortable in as well as being smart and present yourself well. Good preparation is crucial to your success. This may include finding out about what research is being carried out within the institution and who is leading on different areas of research; or learning how to conduct research, the underlying principles and methods of analysis. If the position is more strategic, you may need to read and be able to summarise relevant policy documents. For those involved in the selection process it is evident who has prepared (even if they are nervous), and who is unprepared and unsure. Finally, when in the interview, listen to the question being asked and take your time to answer succinctly.

KEY POINTS

It is for us as members of the nursing profession to acknowledge relevant research within our fields of practice, and to take into consideration the following key points:

 Plan your career; do not let it happen by chance or by somebody else's whim.

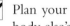 Review all post-registration courses and pick those most relevant to your practice and career development.

 Base your practice on sound research evidence; if there are important gaps in knowledge raise awareness of this so that relevant research is undertaken.

 Collaborate with colleagues; nurses need to work together to take the profession forward.

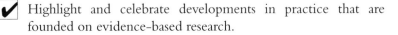 Highlight and celebrate developments in practice that are founded on evidence-based research.

REFERENCES

Baly, M.E. (1980) *Nursing and Social Change*, 2nd edition. London: Heinemann.

Committee on Nursing (1972) *Report of the Committee of Nursing (Briggs Report)*. London: Committee on Nursing.

Department of Health (1999) *Making a Difference. Strengthening the Nursing, Midwifery and Health Visiting Contribution to Health and Healthcare*. London: Department of Health.

Weir, R. (1996) *A Leap in the Dark: The Origins and Development of the Department of Nursing Studies at the University of Edinburgh*. London: Book Factory.

CAREERS IN RESEARCH

Index

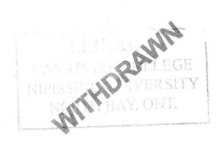